MW00389405

The Intensive Care Unit: What Every Family Needs to Know

STEVEN R. MOHNSSEN, M.D.

Robert D. Reed Publishers   San Francisco, CA

Copyright © 2001 by Steven R. Mohnssen, M. D.
All rights reserved.

No part of this book may be reproduced without written permission from the publisher or copyright holder, except for a reviewer who may quote brief passages in a review. Nor may any part of this book be reproduced, stored in a retrieval system, or transmitted in any form or by any means electronic, mechanical, photocopying, recording or other, without written permission from the publisher or copyright holder.

Disclaimer: This book is written for educational purposes only, and the author is not engaged in rendering medical advice or recommendations. Since this book is not a substitute for medical advice or treatment, the author recommends consultation with your physician or qualified health care professional for your individual medical needs.

Robert D. Reed Publishers
750 La Playa Street, Suite 647
San Francisco, CA 94121
Phone: 650/994-6570 • Fax: -6579
E-mail: 4bobreed@msn.com
www.rdrpublishers.com

Editor: Margaret Duggar
Book Designer: Marilyn Yasmine Nadel
Cover Designer: Julia Gaskill

ISBN 1-885003-95-1

Library of Congress Control Number: 2001090960

Produced and Printed in the United States of America

*I would like to dedicate this book
first to my loving family:
my beautiful wife Vicki
and my children, Carter and Ashley,
who patiently tolerated the countless hours
required to complete this project in my spare time.*

*Second, I want to express my gratitude to my parents,
Ray and Sue,
for they encouraged me when I showed
an interest in writing as a child.*

Table of Contents

Foreword

As a hospital chaplain, I have been with many patients and their families as they face the ICU (Intensive Care Unit) and Emergency Room experience. In my role as chaplain, my primary focus is to help people find spiritual and emotional comfort as they face difficult life situations. For many, the sudden trip to an Emergency Room or ICU is like going to a strange and frightening country. This book is a sort of travel guide, explaining the lay of the land where the natives (doctors, nurses and therapy specialists) often use strange words and unintelligible abbreviations. This is a book that will help to translate that 'foreign language'. (The Glossary of Common Medical Terms at the end, in itself is worth the price.)

This book comes at a fitting time in the continuing evolution of medical care. During the last thirty or so years I have witnessed many developments which especially call forth the need for a new guide like this:

—There has been a remarkable growth and sophistication in the technological support of our patients. More than ever, when we enter and ICU we are shocked to see our loved ones connected up to a bewildering array of tubes, needles, wires, pumps, monitors (which beep and sound alarms) and other devices. These can give us the feeling of entering a "Twilight Zone" of science fiction. To some it can feel cold, impersonal and frightening. We may wonder where all the warm, hands-on caring has gone.

—New diagnostic, medical and surgical procedures continue to be invented. Thankfully, the goal is to do even more effective procedures less invasively than they were done in the past. Early in my career, CAT scans (Computed Aided Tomography), MRIs (Magnetic Resonance Imaging) and many kinds of microsurgery were unknown. These often require a lot of interpretation for patients and families

—In the past there was a passive "Doctor knows best" attitude. Now legal requirements are moving doctor-patient relationships to greater informed consent. The medical staff bears more responsibility to educate patients and family about various procedures and options, and the recipients of medical care carry more responsibility to learn about medical options and to make difficult decisions. (In the '60's there were no DPAHC [Durable Power of Attorney for Health Care] legal documents, nor were DNR [Do Not Resuscitate] orders well known and used.) There is now greater public awareness of high tech care, often from TV's "E.R." and other medical shows. These can both inform and sometimes, confuse the issues.

—Medical/financial realities have changed. With the ever-tightening fiscal constraints doctors, nurses and hospitals are faced with, there is a change in the relationship and time that a doctor has with his/her patients and their families. Nurses and other health care providers also have less time to educate and explain procedures.

The issues that arise in ICU and Emergency medical situations often cause us to think and feel deep thoughts and emotions that are at the core of our humanity and our relationships with our loved ones. I therefore see the ICU/ER as a deeply human place.

One additional comment: I am aware that many people see all these changes and advances as 'cold technology'. Over the years I have witnessed the caring, warmth and inventiveness on the part of medical people that is behind these technologies. I am personally grateful. On December 14th, 1996, I had a heart attack. While on a monitored gurney going from the Emergency Room to the Catheterization Lab, I went "flat line" (heart stopped) seven times. Because of the technology and the skill of three cardiac nurses I was resuscitated an equal number of times. Under the skilled care of my cardiologist and the Cath Lab staff and through the wonders of balloon angioplasty I woke up to their cheers. I now enjoy a full and active life. For me, "high tech" is truly "warm tech" and I am grateful.

As you tour the land of ICU/ER I would hope you will have moments where you will let your jaw drop at the wonders of modern medicine and your eyes raise in gratitude for the rich resources available to us and those we love. I believe this book will help you to do both.

As a chaplain, I am concerned about the relational and spiritual wellbeing of patients and families. I am convinced that being able to understand what is happening and to communicate clearly with each other and with medical personnel are some of the most effective ways of finding peace and comfort, and making wise, caring decisions. I therefore champion this book and commend it to you.

Rev. Walter E. Johnson, M. Div.
San Mateo, California

Preface

This book was written as a guide for you, as a family member or friend of someone who has been admitted to one of the hospital "intensive care" or "critical care" units. These specialized hospital units or wards provide care for patients who are critically ill and suffering from a wide variety of medical and surgical illnesses. Most commonly, abbreviations are used to describe certain types of intensive care units, depending on the type of patients cared for in that particular unit. For example, those with "medical" illnesses such as severe infections, pneumonia, breathing problems, etc., are often admitted either to an ICU (intensive care unit) or MICU (medical intensive care unit). In some cases, specialized intensive care units exist for certain surgical specialties such as SICU (surgical intensive care unit), NICU (neurosurgical intensive care unit), CCU (cardiac care unit) and others.

As a physician specializing in pulmonary disease and critical care medicine, I have learned firsthand that families and friends of patients who are being cared for in an ICU have many questions about their loved one's illness and their ICU experience. These questions and concerns are wide ranging but often center around the disease process itself, prognosis and severity of the illness, expectations and treatment options, concerns about equipment, monitoring devices, procedures, and visiting hours. Unquestionably, visiting a loved one at the bedside or maintaining a vigil in the intensive care waiting room can be a frightening and emotional experience.

I believe that you will be able to cope more effectively if you are provided with a reasonable amount of information about your loved one's disease and treatment in easily understood language. Unfortunately, the usual combination of fear, anxiety, and sleep deprivation may make it understandably difficult for you to absorb all of the information that is provided to you by your physician or nurse. Despite their best intentions, health care providers may not be able to give you all the informational support you need due to the demands of their health care responsibilities.

This publication attempts to supplement the important information that may have already been provided to you by your physician and other health care providers. It can serve as a basic introduction to the ICU experience and provide a simple background to common disease processes, enabling you to review the material at a leisurely pace. It should be emphasized that this book does not include a full description of each disease, but instead provides basic background material. This material will not provide specific treatment guidelines on any disease process, as that information can only be obtained directly from the physician or health care provider involved in the daily care of the critically ill patient. Only your physician knows the best treatment plan for your loved one.

The idea for this book came to me after one of my discussions with a family in an intensive care unit waiting room. After twelve years of practicing critical care medicine, it became clear to me that these people need a convenient and easy to read resource to refer to in order to help answer the questions that often remain after discussions with their physician(s). If you have specific questions about a disease, medical procedure, or treatment, this book provides a quick reference. In addition, the Glossary/Index in the back of the book is useful if you are having trouble understanding some of the medical terms you may hear during your discussions with physicians and other health care providers. Even if you don't have specific questions, I suggest that you read the first three chapters of the book as important background material, then skip to the appropriate chapter(s) that cover the disease process that you are interested in. At the end of each chapter is a blank page that is available for you to write questions or take notes for your next discussion with a physician or nurse.

Steven R. Mohnssen, MD

Acknowledgments

From the idea stage to publication, this book took nearly three years to complete. I especially wish to acknowledge the following people who have proven invaluable to me while writing this book:

Margaret Duggar, who proved that she is an excellent editor and an indispensable resource to any writer.

Julia Gaskill, whose creative talents are displayed on the book cover.

Marilyn Yasmine Nadel, who provided her layout/design expertise, and was willing to respond promptly to deadline requests and multiple text changes.

Rev. Walter Johnson, whose words of wisdom and genuine kindness will not be forgotten.

The support given by the intensive care unit staff at Columbus Regional Hospital, Columbus, Indiana.

Chapter One
Monitors, Signals
and Visiting Hours

Monitors

It is essential to monitor changes in the condition of a critically ill patient. For example, if the blood pressure or heart rate drops too low or rises too high, or the blood oxygen level drops too low, this may tell the health care provider to change therapies. In addition, it suggests the need to look into the reason for the change in the patients' condition. The technology for monitoring patients is very sensitive and effective, and will produce sound signals when the vital sign being monitored becomes "out of range." Unfortunately, the many signals, beeps and noises heard in the intensive care unit can be quite frightening and anxiety-provoking for family members when they are visiting their loved ones.

The most common vital signs that need to be monitored at the bedside include blood pressure, heart rate and rhythm, pulse oximetry (blood oxygen level), and respiratory rate (how fast a person is breathing). Most of the monitoring devices have pre-programmed or manually set ranges for "normal" and "abnormal," and when these ranges are exceeded a signal will sound.

Many of these vital signs will show as a "waveform" (a line that goes up and down like a "wave" or "blip") that can be seen on a screen near the patients' bed. Remember that some of these waveforms can be occasionally flat or almost flat, even though nothing has changed for the worse with regard to the patient. When the patient requires more intensive monitoring or testing, more waveforms can be added and others can be replaced as needed on the bedside monitor. These more complex monitoring devices may include pulmonary artery catheters or "Swan-Ganz" catheters, arterial catheters or "art" lines, CVP catheters (central venous pressure lines), and others.

Sound Signals

One of the more frequent causes of sound signals in the intensive care unit is the mechanical ventilator. A ventilator is a machine that is placed next to the bedside and is used to "breathe" for a patient who can't breathe well enough on his/her own. Commonly, when the machine is turned on and is breathing for the patient, signals within the ventilator may sound for many reasons. For example, a ventilator signal may sound when an individual is coughing, causing the high-pressure signal to go off until the cough stops. Signals may also occur when the respiratory care practitioner is adjusting the ventilator, manipulating the tubing from the ventilator to the patient, or suctioning mucous from the patients' airway.

Since there are wide ranges in "normal" vital sign values in individual patients who may have differing illnesses, it may not be a good idea to concentrate on the numbers displayed on the monitor when visiting a patient. If you pay too much attention to specific numbers on the monitor, the frequent and continuous changes may cause you undue stress and concern. While there certainly are times when a sound signal may mean the patient is having an emergency to which the medical staff will immediately respond, the usual situation is that there is nothing to worry about, and the health care providers are aware of the signals, what they mean, and how to respond. In general, most of the sounds heard in the intensive care unit do not mean that there is an emergency occurring.

One way to reduce anxiety about monitoring systems and

their signals is for you to take a brief "guided tour" (if time allows) of the bedside monitor system with the nursing staff when your friend or loved one has been admitted to the intensive care unit. At the same time, you can review the ventilator and its expected signals with the respiratory care practitioner. This discussion will prove valuable to you, the family member or friend, and provide reassurance during a difficult time.

Visiting Hours

Visiting a family member who is stricken with a serious illness can be a frightening experience. It is important to realize that patients need the support of their family, and this support plays an important role in the recovery process. Most intensive care units have visiting hours designed to provide you this important time with your loved one. However, critically ill patients have only a limited amount of strength and energy, and they may tire easily if visitors are constantly at the bedside, even though the visitors have good intentions.

"Non-visiting hours" were therefore created by intensive care unit staff in order to provide critically ill patients with the time for essential rest and healing and also so that the nursing staff and other health care providers will have the time to examine, treat, and provide important patient care.

It is advisable during your "guided tour" to review with the nursing staff the posted visiting hours so that there will be less chance of confusion or frustration. In addition, the individual nurse assigned to your loved one can give you guidance on how to most effectively communicate with and support your loved one.

Unquestionably, the signals, machines, and monitors in the ICU can be intimidating during your ICU visits. However, once you have a basic understanding of what they mean, why they exist, and how the staff will use them, your visits to the ICU will be a little less anxiety provoking.

Notes and Questions for the Doctor, Nurse, or
Respiratory Care Practitioner:

Chapter Two
Nutrition, Lines, and Medications

Intravenous Lines

When visiting your loved one in the intensive care unit, you will commonly see multiple lines, tubes and wires attached to the patient.

Intravenous lines (IV's) are very small pliable plastic tubes or "catheters" which are inserted into the veins of the arms in order to provide fluids, blood products, nutrition and certain medications. Tubing from these lines is commonly connected to an IV bottle or bag, which is hanging from a pole next to the bed. Medications can be given through these intravenous lines. Often medications can be infused directly, or by a "piggyback" bag, which hangs on the IV pole next to the fluid bag, and allows the medication to drip slowly into the patient's vein with the fluid. When given into the bloodstream directly by the intravenous route, these medications will work quicker than when given by mouth, and it is not unusual for patients in the ICU to be unable to take medications by mouth.

On occasions when the patient does not have veins in the arms that are easy to access, a large amount of fluid or blood must be infused quickly, or high calorie intravenous feedings become necessary, a "central line" may need to be placed. A central line is basically a larger diameter and longer IV catheter that has several additional access ports attached, therefore allowing larger amounts of fluid and multiple medications to be given together into a larger vein. These central lines are placed by the physician into one of the larger veins located either under the collar bone (subclavian line), the internal or external jugular vein in the neck, or the femoral vein in the groin area. These catheters are put in under a local anesthetic and often with sedative medications as well, for the comfort of the patient. A "Swan-Ganz" pulmonary artery catheter is similar to a central line, yet more complex. Physicians use the same technique to gain access to the large veins when inserting central lines and pulmonary artery catheters. However, with pulmonary artery catheters, an "introducer" is placed as a central line access to one of the large veins in the neck or under the collarbone. A soft, flexible catheter with several ports and a tip that allows inflation of a small balloon is then inserted through the introducer. The balloon is inflated, then advanced by "flotation" in the blood stream into the right atrium of the heart, right ventricle, then into the pulmonary artery where it can be temporarily "wedged" to obtain valuable pressure measurements. Physicians use these pressure measurements to determine the volume and pressure that the heart generates, as well as the cardiac output or "horsepower" of the heart. The information they provide is useful in calculating fluid balance and the need for medications in certain critically ill individuals. While these procedures are generally safe, the potential advantages as well as complications of any such procedure are best discussed with your physician.

Nutrition

Although nutrition can be provided by the IV method, the best method of feeding is by mouth. However, it is not unusual to find very ill individuals who are unable to feed themselves by mouth due to the fact that they may be connected to the ventilator machine (See Chapter 3). In addition, they may be too sleepy due to their illness or suffer from an abdominal disease that prevents ordinary eating.

Feedings can be given through small tubes that are inserted into the nose and passed into the esophagus (swallowing tube) then into the stomach (N-G tube), or they can be inserted by way of the mouth and then into the stomach (O-G tube). If the feedings are needed for a long time, a surgeon or gastroen-terologist may be asked to place a tube surgically from the skin of the abdomen into either the stomach (G-tube, PEG tube, or gastrostomy tube), or into a portion of the small intestine. (Jejunostomy tube or J-tube) Various liquid nutritional products can be infused into these feeding tubes in order to provide nutritional support to patients. Vitamins as well as liquid medications can also be given via these feeding tubes.

Total Parenteral Nutrition

When feedings cannot be provided into the stomach or small intestine by mouth, or all the calorie needs of the patient cannot be met using a feeding tube, total parenteral nutrition (TPN) may become necessary. TPN is a method of feeding that uses complex formulations of specially prepared nutrients (amino acids, sugars, fatty acids, vitamins and minerals) and infuses them into a central line IV. Due to the high concentrations of sugars that can be in these formulations, blood sugar measurements may be necessary. If blood sugar levels rise too high while on TPN, insulin may need to be added to the TPN bag, or the patient may require insulin injections. These high blood sugar levels are usually temporary and resolve or improve after the TPN is removed. TPN is usually considered as a short-term feeding method, until it becomes possible to use the digestive system directly.

Clearly, nutrition is important and you can be reassured that if your loved one is not able to eat in the usual way, there are several other methods of feeding other than by mouth. In addition, I have described several different types and "styles" of intravenous lines, depending on patient need. Although you will see multiple different tubes and lines in the ICU, if there is one that you don't understand, please don't hesitate to ask your nurse or physician.

Suggested Resources for Additional Information:

The American Dietetic Association
Website: www.eatright.org

Medline Plus Health Information
"Nutritional Support"
Website: www.nlm.nih/medlineplus/nutritional support

Notes and Questions for the Doctor or Nurse:

_____

_____

_____

_____

_____

_____

_____

_____

_____

_____

_____

_____

_____

_____

_____

_____

_____

_____

_____

_____

_____

_____

_____

_____

_____

_____

_____

Chapter Three

The Ventilator

When we breathe, the lungs remove oxygen from the air and then supply it to the blood stream. In addition, the lungs remove the waste product CO2 (carbon dioxide) from the blood stream.

A ventilator is a machine that provides breathing assistance to a patient who is having severe difficulty breathing. Ventilators provide oxygen, but in addition, they also provide a volume of air or air pressure, which automatically expands the lungs and does the breathing for the patient. These machines give the patient a "rest" from the hard work of breathing. It is important to note that many people who have trouble breathing and who have low blood oxygen levels may need only oxygen supplied through a simple nasal cannula or oxygen mask only, without the requirement for a ventilator machine. Low to moderate concentrations of oxygen can be supplied by a nasal cannula or mask; however, the ventilator can accurately provide a range of oxygen concentration from (21% (room air) up to 100%). Only when the breathing trouble becomes severe does it become necessary to remove the nasal cannula or oxygen mask and proceed to place the patient on the ventilator machine. Most commonly, this occurs when the individual has an oxygen level in the blood that is too low to be adequately corrected by a mask or nasal oxygen source, the CO_2 level in the blood is becoming too high, or the patient is using too much energy to breathe and is showing signs of fatigue. Depending on the condition of the patient, a ventilator may only be necessary for a day or two, or it may be in place for multiple days, weeks or longer.

The most common reason for a patient to require a ventilator machine is respiratory failure. Although lung diseases are the most common causes of respiratory failure, many other illnesses can cause the patient to develop respiratory failure and therefore require the ventilator machine. A brief list of these illnesses includes: severe pneumonia, COPD (chronic obstructive pulmonary disease), shock due to severe infection in the bloodstream (sepsis), poisoning, drug overdoses, stroke or other neurologic diseases (ALS or amyotrophic lateral sclerosis, myasthenia gravis, muscular dystrophy etc.), pulmonary embolism (blood clots in the lungs), traumatic brain injury, respiratory difficulty after surgical procedures and many others. For further details on specific disease processes, please see the Glossary/Index.

In order to connect the patient to the ventilator, physicians and health care providers place endotracheal tubes in the mouth or through the nostril into the trachea (windpipe), which then provides direct access to the lungs. The endotracheal tube then resides midway in the trachea while the patient remains on the ventilator. During the process of inserting the endotracheal tube, the physician will order medications that will make the individual sleepy and help relieve discomfort. While the ventilator is connected to the end of the endotracheal tube and expanding the patients' lungs, he or she will not be able to talk. If the patient is awake, this may require writing pads or other methods to help with communication. Additional medications will be available for the comfort of the patient while on the ventilator machine, and many of these medications will cause sleepiness, and therefore, your loved one may be difficult to arouse at times. In addition, for the sake of safety, wrist restraints may be necessary so that the patient doesn't accidentally remove the lines or tubes.

When an endotracheal tube resides in the trachea, the patient will be unable to adequately cough to expel mucous. Therefore, your loved one may require "suctioning" intermittently while on the ventilator. In order to "suction" the patient, nursing or respiratory staff pass a soft, flexible catheter down the endotracheal tube and suction secretions as needed.

Tracheostomy

If the ventilator is required for a relatively long period (anywhere from one to two weeks or more), some gradual injury may occur to the vocal cords or windpipe, although this may not happen, and is hard to predict. At a certain point during a long stay in the ICU on a ventilator, your physician may discuss with you the possibility of providing your loved one with a"tracheostomy" tube. A tracheostomy tube is a tube that can be placed surgically using an incision on the front of the neck below the voice box into the trachea (windpipe). This device helps by allowing continued use of the ventilator, with less risk of damaging the vocal cords. Certainly the advantages and disadvantages of tracheostomy should be discussed with your physician. Please note that there is not a standard, "best" time when a tracheostomy should be placed, and that this is clearly a decision made by the physician according to the patients' needs.

Blood Gases And Pulse Oximetry

As discussed in chapter 1, oxygen levels are frequently monitored when a patient is on the ventilator. This can be done with a blood sample taken from a wrist artery, called an "arterial blood gas" This will accurately measure blood oxygen (O_2), carbon dioxide (CO_2), and pH (acid level in the blood). In addition, "pulse oximetry" is a widely used way of continuously monitoring oxygen levels. With pulse oximetry, a probe is painlessly placed like a loosely fitting clamp on the finger or ear lobe. It is then able to estimate the blood oxygen level and record it on a monitor. Pulse oximetry does not provide as much information as the arterial blood gas, but is nevertheless very valuable in monitoring changes in blood oxygen levels. An added benefit of pulse oximetry is that it is less invasive then a blood gas, does not require a needle puncture, and does not cause pain.

Ventilator Weaning and Liberation

While on the ventilator, your health care providers will use terms such as "weaning" from the ventilator and "liberation" from the ventilator. This means that the physician believes that the patient has improved enough to allow removal of the ventilator machine, and therefore the endotracheal tube can be removed also. Several techniques are commonly used for weaning, and they depend on the specific situation and the physician's analysis of the patient's capabilities. Whichever weaning technique is chosen, the patient will need to be alert and cooperative during the process. This will require that the physician discontinue or perhaps reduce the amount of sleep-provoking medicines that the individual receives. One method of weaning requires the patient to keep the breathing tube in, but the ventilator no longer provides mandatory "breaths" to the individual. Instead, the ventilator provides oxygen and small amounts of "pressure support." This means the patient is breathing on his or her own, and if he/ she does well during the trial, the tube may be removed from the patient, and the ventilator is no longer needed. This method of weaning is called the "T-tube" trial or "CPAP" trial.

Another method of removal from the ventilator requires a gradual reduction in the breaths that are delivered by the ventilator. This allows the patient to show his/her ability to breathe without as many machine breaths. For example, if the patient is getting all of his/her breaths from the ventilator, his/her body may not need to take any additional breaths on its own. If the ventilator is providing twelve breaths per minute, the ventilator can then be turned down to provide only six breaths per minute, and the individual will now be allowed to breathe on his/her own in between the ventilator breaths, thus providing a total of twelve breaths or more per minute. The number of ventilator breaths will gradually be reduced to zero, and then the individual will be breathing completely without help from the machine.

There is no "best" method for liberation from the ventilator, however, whichever method the physician chooses, the patient will likely need oxygen after extubation (removal of breathing tube), using either a nasal cannula or mask.

Hoarseness is not uncommon after removing the breathing tube, and the patient will likely be talking again some time later, often within thirty to sixty minutes. Patients are not pushed to begin talking until they feel rested and comfortable enough to do so. Not uncommonly, it may also take several hours or longer until an individual will be able to safely and comfortably drink liquids or even try to eat soft foods.

This chapter provided an introduction to a very complex piece of equipment - the ventilator. Hopefully you will now have a little more understanding of how these machines work, why your loved one may need one, what procedures are necessary to place the patient on the ventilator, and why blood gases and oximetry are important. This knowledge will serve you well as you listen to your physician, nurse, or respiratory therapist as they provide daily progress reports.

Suggested Resources for Additional Information:

The American Lung Association
Website: www. Lungusa.org
Address: 1740 Broadway, NY, NY, 10019
Phone: 1-800-Lung-USA (1-800-586-4872)

Notes and Questions for the Doctor, Nurse, or
Respiratory Care Practitioner:

Chapter Four
Diseases of the Lung

COPD

Chronic obstructive pulmonary disease (COPD) is a broad term used for several similar diseases including chronic bronchitis, emphysema, bronchiectasis and asthma. These diseases are similar in that they all are associated with obstruction to airflow when breathing out, either due to blockage by mucous or by spasm of the smooth muscle that surrounds the bronchial passages (breathing tubes) in the lungs. Either way, the patient will develop symptoms due to the narrowing of the bronchial tubes. Commonly, patients with COPD will have difficulty with breathing, wheezing, coughing, and in some cases, abnormalities in their arterial blood gas measurements (see Chapter 3). Bronchodilator medicines (inhaled medications) are frequently provided to these patients in order to open the narrowed bronchial tubes caused by smooth muscle spasm. In addition, the patient's doctor may prescribe steroids and various oral, inhaled, and intravenous medications.

If the patient with COPD does not improve with the medications described above and becomes severely breathless and fatigued, or supplemental oxygen by mask or nasal cannula is not successful in providing adequate amounts of oxygen in the blood, the patient may have to be placed on a ventilator machine (see Chapter 3).

Pneumonia

Pneumonia is an infection in one or both lungs. This infection can reside in a small area (segment), a larger area (lobe), or it may involve several areas of both lungs in more severe cases. Pneumonia can often be seen on chest x-rays, and may be preceded by a persistent cough, fever, or trouble breathing. Most commonly pneumonia is caused by bacteria, but it may also be caused by viruses, fungi, parasites or other organisms. Antibiotics and other appropriate anti-infective medications are given to the patient in order to fight the infection. Cultures of blood and respiratory secretions may be necessary in some cases in order to guide treatment. Severe pneumonias may result in difficulty breathing and low blood oxygen levels despite the fact that the patient is receiving supplemental oxygen. In some of these cases, your physician may need to place your loved one on the ventilator while treatment continues (see Chapter 3).

Adult Respiratory Distress Syndrome (ARDS)

ARDS is a condition of the lungs that always requires that the patient be placed on the ventilator in order to improve severely reduced blood oxygen levels. In this condition, the lung becomes "injured" from a variety of causes, and damage to the lining or the air sacs (alveoli) and capillaries (small blood vessels) cause fluid, protein, and other substances to leak into the lung tissue itself. This fluid accumulation in the lungs is called pulmonary edema, and is seen fairly easily on chest x-rays. The pulmonary edema that happens in ARDS is different from the fluid that builds up due to heart failure. Unfortunately, it may be more difficult to remove fluid from the "injured" lung of ARDS than from the "normal" lung seen in heart failure. The causes of ARDS are many: traumatic injuries, severe pneumonia, pancreatitis, burns, septic shock, inhalation of toxic gas or chemicals, aspiration of stomach acid, and others. Clearly ARDS is a serious disease process, which requires aggressive treatment and complex ventilator management techniques in the intensive care unit.

Pulmonary Embolus

A pulmonary embolus is a blood clot that travels from veins in the leg or pelvis into the lung blood vessels (pulmonary arteries) and causes shortness of breath, chest discomfort, and often times, low blood oxygen levels. Tests are available to help the physician with this sometimes-difficult diagnosis, and the physician may treat the individual with "blood-thinning" medications. Although pulmonary emboli usually don't cause the patient to be placed on the ventilator, large clots that cause severe illness may require the ventilator for patient support.

Pneumothorax

Pneumothorax is a condition that occurs when air leaks into the pleural cavity. (The pleural cavity is the narrow space between the lung and the rib cage). This can occur from a variety of causes. Depending on the size of the "air leak," a pneumothorax may or may not be associated with symptoms of breathlessness or chest discomfort. A small pneumothorax may be observed over time and may resolve without treatment. However, a larger pneumothorax, or one that causes significant symptoms, may require placement of a chest tube or catheter through the skin and over a rib into the pleural space in order to remove the unwanted air pocket. Chest tubes can be placed at the bedside under local anesthesia with medications that keep the patient comfortable and in less pain.

Atelectasis

Atelectasis is a term that refers to a condition whereby a portion of the lung, or the whole lung itself, may "collapse." This is similar to your attempting to "blow-up" a balloon that is partially pinched at the opening: some air is allowed to go in, but the balloon can only be partly expanded, and does not achieve maximum size. Most commonly, atelectasis occurs when patients don't take deep enough breaths after surgery, or when a plug of mucous or a solid mass obstructs the airflow to one of the breathing tubes in the lung. Atelectasis is usually diagnosed on X-rays of the chest, and may cause difficulty breathing, low blood oxygen levels, and a predisposition to pneumonia. Multiple methods are available to treat this common condition. A brief list of some of these methods includes: taking deep breaths with a device called an "incentive spirometer," breathing inhaled medications to "open-up" closed airways, and forced coughing. Sometimes bronchoscopy may become necessary in order to physically remove mucous plugs.

Pleural Effusions And Empyemas

A pleural effusion is an abnormal collection of fluid that accumulates in the pleural cavity. Pleural effusions can occur due to many conditions: trauma, pneumonia, pulmonary emboli, heart failure, cancer and others. Most often, these effusions are thin and "free-flowing," and if they are causing symptoms such as breathlessness or chest discomfort, they can be drained with simple needle drainage under local anesthesia (thoracentesis) and/or the disease that causes the fluid can be treated so that the pleural effusion improves. However, when the pleural fluid becomes severely infected, the fluid can become thick and acidic, causing chest discomfort, breathlessness, and fever despite the use of appropriate antibiotics. This condition is called empyema. Often empyemas occur in association with pneumonias, although not all pneumonias cause empyema. Initially, a thoracentesis may be done in order to make the diagnosis and to set up cultures and other lab tests as necessary. If the thoracentesis is not successful in draining the pleural fluid, a chest tube may become necessary in order to complete the drainage of the infected fluid. If the empyema is extremely thick and acidic, it may form a "peel" around the lung, which can't be drained by a needle or tube. In this situation, your physician may consider surgical options to remove the infection and the "peel." Antibiotics will most likely be given in conjunction with these drainage procedures.

Chest Trauma and Surgery

Traumatic injuries to the chest, due to their severity and life-threatening potential, may require immediate surgery (thoracotomy or median sternotomy). These patients will need close monitoring in the intensive care unit and may require the ventilator machine for breathing support, blood transfusions to replace blood loss (see Chapter 10), chest tubes to drain blood from the pleural cavity or to treat pneumothorax, central lines for intravenous access, and sometimes "Swan-Ganz" pulmonary artery catheters for fluid and heart pressure monitoring (see Chapter 2).

Lung Transplantation

The first human lung transplant was performed in 1963. Early on, the results were disappointing until advances were made in drug therapy for organ rejection in the 1980's, and therefore lung transplants became much more common in the 1990's. Some of the more common diseases that may be considered for lung transplant include: COPD, alpha-1 antitrypsin deficiency, emphysema, idiopathic pulmonary fibrosis, cystic fibrosis, primary pulmonary hypertension, and others. Certainly lung transplantation is a major procedure and not all patients with the above conditions are good candidates for it.

After the transplant, the patient will be moved to the ICU immediately. Early after surgery, the major problems that can occur are mostly due to infections and graft failure (failure of the donor lung). After the first month, problems commonly can occur due to the patient's immune system attempting to "reject" the donor lung, and also due to possible problems with infections.

In the ICU after a transplant, the patient will require the ventilator machine, and it will be "weaned" off as the patient improves. Immunosuppressive drugs (drugs that reduce the body's ability to fight off invading substances) will be started either just before or after surgery in order to combat the natural tendency of the body to "reject" or destroy the donor organ. Unfortunately, these drugs may themselves cause the patient to be vulnerable to infections such as bacteria, fungi, and viruses. Commonly, antibiotics will be used both to prevent and treat these infections. The ICU team will pay close attention to fluid balance, blood pressure, and other vital signs. Monitoring for the possibility of rejection and infection may require bronchoscopy (a bronchoscope is a flexible tube with a light that is used to provide cultures as well as lung biopsies).

Although this chapter provides only brief descriptions of a few of the many diseases that can involve the lungs, a good background knowledge of these common conditions may be helpful, because they are seen in almost every ICU on a daily basis.

Suggested Resources for Additional Information:

The American Lung Association
1740 Broadway, NY, NY 10019
Phone: 1 800-Lung-USA
Website: www.Lungusa.org

National Asthma Education Program Information Center
4733 Bethesda Ave., suite 530
Bethesda, Md. 20814
Phone: 301-951-3260

The Society of Thoracic Surgeons
401 N. Michigan Ave..
Chicago, Il 60611-4267
Website: www.sts.org (look under "patient information")
Phone 312-644-6610

Notes and Questions for the Doctor, Nurse, or Respiratory Care Practitioner:

Chapter Five

Diseases of the Heart

Angina

Angina (pronounced AN-ji-nah or an-JI-nah) is an uncomfortable or painful feeling that occurs in a patient's chest, jaw, back, arm or neck. Other symptoms include heaviness or tingling in arms, elbows, and wrists, as well as nausea, indigestion and difficulty breathing. If your loved one is experiencing this type of discomfort, it is possible that his/her heart may not be getting enough oxygen-rich blood to perform properly. Certainly there are other causes of this type of discomfort, but it is important to evaluate the patient for heart disease first. Angina is not a heart attack, but it is a symptom of heart disease. Angina often occurs during exertion or emotional stress, and goes away with medicines or rest. If the angina discomfort lasts longer or starts occurring more often, then it is called "unstable angina."

Angina is a symptom of a type of heart disease called coronary artery disease. Basically, coronary artery disease is a condition that occurs when the blood vessels supplying blood to the heart muscle become clogged with a fatty material called plaque. The clogged arteries will then supply less oxygen and blood to the muscle, especially during exertion and stress, thus causing angina. The risks for coronary artery disease include smoking, high cholesterol, high blood pressure, lack of exercise, strong family history of cardiac disease, and diabetes.

Physicians diagnose angina with various tests, depending on the situation. This may include EKG (electrocardiogram) performed at rest and during exercise (stress test), echocardiogram (ultrasound machine that bounces sound waves off the heart to provide a picture of the heart chambers), stress echocardiogram, nuclear scans, and angiograms (cardiac catheterization). A cardiac catheterization is a thin, flexible tube that is inserted into an artery in the arm or groin, and then guided into the heart. Discomfort is minimized with local "numbing medicine" and sedative medication. Dye is released, and X-rays will show the details of the blood flow in the coronary arteries. These catheterizations are performed in special cardiac catheterization labs, and usually do not require the patient to be in the ICU after the procedure, unless complications occur.

Multiple medications are available for treatment as well as prevention of angina. Your physician will decide what is the best treatment depending on the individual situation.

Acute Myocardial Infarction (Heart Attack)

Heart attacks happen when blood flow through a coronary artery (blood vessel that supplies blood and oxygen to the heart muscle) suddenly stops because a clot forms inside the artery. This reduced blood flow to the heart muscle (ischemia) causes damage to the heart muscle, which worsens as time passes unless the blood flow improves. Medicines are available that can restore blood flow by dissolving the clot that has formed in one or more of the coronary arteries. It is important, however, that the patient be brought to the nearest emergency facility as soon as possible so that the clot-dissolving drugs can be given quickly after symptoms occur. These medicines are not as effective if treatment is delayed too long; time is clearly very important.

Heart attack patients are brought from the emergency department to the ICU or Coronary Care Unit so that they can be observed closely during and after treatment, and also to quickly identify and treat any complications. Complications can include abnormal electrical heart rhythms such as ventricular fibrillation or ventricular tachycardia, congestive heart failure (reduced "pumping" ability of the heart muscle), and shock (severely reduced blood pressure).

After the heart attack patient has stabilized and improved, other procedures may or may not be necessary. These procedures may include balloon angioplasty (small balloon is inflated at the end of a catheter which is advanced into a narrowed coronary artery), coronary stents (a coil or mesh is placed into the coronary artery to keep it open), or sometimes surgical procedures such as coronary artery bypass surgery may be recommended by your family member's physician in order to increase blood flow to the heart muscle.

Coronary Bypass Surgery (CABG)

Coronary artery bypass surgery is a relatively frequently performed heart operation. There are a variety of reasons why this surgery may be recommended: life threatening blockage of a coronary artery, complications after a heart attack, or failure of medications to resolve angina (chest pain). Not everyone is a candidate for surgery, and your physician will determine this.

The goal of this surgery is to provide a detour around the blocked coronary arteries in order to supply more oxygen and blood flow to the heart muscle itself. Before surgery, a cardiac catheterization will be performed so the physician can locate which arteries need to be "bypassed." A cardiac catheterization involves the insertion of a thin flexible tube (catheter) into a groin artery that is then passed into the heart. Dye is injected through the catheter, and the anatomy of your coronary arteries as well as the heart's pumping action and valve function can then be seen on an X-ray monitor.

Bypass surgery itself can last from two to six hours depending on the number of bypass grafts required. An incision is made into the breastbone, which is divided to allow access to the heart. Other, less invasive techniques may be possible at some institutions. Veins form the patient's leg or the internal mammary artery may be removed (as they are not essential to the body) and can be used to bypass or detour around the obstructed heart arteries.

After surgery, patients will be monitored in the intensive care unit during their recovery. The patient will have multiple tubes after surgery, including an endotracheal tube (see Chapter 3), bladder catheter, intravenous lines, arterial catheters, and chest tubes. During recovery, the tubes are gradually removed, and the stay in the ICU will be several days, although individuals do recover at different rates.

Congestive Heart Failure

Congestive heart failure is a common disorder affecting over two million people in the U.S., and up to ten percent of people over the age of 75. In congestive heart failure (CHF), the heart muscle pumps with less force, and therefore the heart chambers stretch and enlarge to hold more blood. Since less blood is pumped, fluid can back up into the lungs, causing "pulmonary edema." Also, less blood flow and therefore less oxygen is provided to other organs such as the kidneys. If the kidneys work less well because of decreased blood supply from the heart, they will not be as effective in removing water, and water may then build up in other areas of the body such as the feet and legs.

CHF occurs as a result of heart attacks, coronary artery disease (narrowing of the heart blood vessels), high blood pressure, heart muscle diseases (cardiomyopathy), and problems with heart valves.

Heart failure can cause shortness of breath, trouble breathing, fatigue, wheezing, and swollen ankles and legs. Shortness of breath is common if the heart failure causes fluid to build up in the lungs. Multiple different treatment options are available for this illness. Most commonly, patients in the intensive care unit who have CHF will have problems with low oxygen levels, shortness of breath, or blood pressure. If oxygen levels or breathing doesn't improve with medications, then the individual may need a ventilator machine until the medications are successful in removing the fluid from the lungs (see Chapter 3 for ventilator discussion).

Heart Transplant

When the heart becomes severely damaged and no longer responds to medicines, a heart transplant may become the best option for certain individuals. With heart transplantation, a healthy donor heart replaces the severely damaged heart.

Heart failure is the usual reason that heart transplants become necessary. Heart failure can occur as a result of coronary artery disease, high blood pressure, heart muscle disease (cardiomyopathy), or other conditions.

Before and after surgery, your loved one will receive extensive evaluation and treatment by a team of experts, including cardiovascular surgeons, cardiologists, nurses, psychologists, infectious disease specialists, social workers, dieticians and chaplains.

Heart transplant patients may require mechanical pumps that help the heart maintain blood circulation (left ventricular assist devices) before the donor heart is transplanted. Immunosuppressive drugs are given either just before or after surgery in order to combat the body's tendency to "reject" the donor organ. Unfortunately, these necessary drugs also make it easier for the transplant patient to get infections, and the transplant team will work hard to prevent them. If infections do occur, a variety of appropriate antibiotics are available for treatment.

After the transplant, the patient will need a ventilator machine in the ICU for a variable period of time, and it will be removed as soon as the patient shows improved strength. A variety of tubes and lines will also be necessary after surgery, in the ICU. These may include, but not be limited to: "Swan-Ganz" pulmonary artery catheters, central lines, arterial lines, bladder catheter, and multiple intravenous medications (see Chapter

2). Once the individual is removed from the ventilator and most of the tubes and lines are removed, the process of rehabilitation can begin.

Aortic Dissection

Aortic dissection refers to a defect in the wall of the aorta (large artery coming from the heart) that allows blood to flow into the layers of tissue that make up the wall of this large artery. The result is a bulging mass that can extend down the aorta and cause significant problems. Patients experience sudden, severe tearing pain in the chest, back or abdomen, often associated with sweating, nausea, or vomiting. This emergency is diagnosed with several tools, including CT scans and transesophageal echocardiograms, depending on what is available in the community. Elevated blood pressure can worsen this condition, and therefore, physicians treat the blood pressure with quick-acting intravenous medicines. Complications can occur from aortic dissection. These may include myocardial infarction (heart attack), stroke, spinal cord or bowel injury, sudden kidney failure, and loss of blood flow to the legs. After the blood pressure is controlled and the diagnosis is made, treatment may be with medicines alone or with surgery, depending on the location and severity of the problem.

Emergencies Due To Hypertension

Some patients are admitted to the ICU because of very high blood pressure. Depending on how severe the problem and the patient's underlying condition, the individual may need aggressive treatment with strong intravenous medications and continuous blood pressure monitoring. This treatment is necessary in order to avoid the harmful effects of the blood pressure on other organs, including the heart, brain (stroke), kidneys, and eyes.

This chapter reviewed some of the major complications that can occur with various heart diseases. You may have noticed that when the heart begins having trouble, other organs become affected also. For example, heart failure can put fluid into the lungs and therefore cause lung trouble (pulmonary edema), and may also cause low blood flow to the kidneys and therefore kidney failure. Obviously, physicians who care for critically ill patients pay close attention to heart function.

Suggested Resources for Additional Information:

American Heart Association
National Center
7272 Greenville Ave.
Dallas, TX 75231
Website: www.americanheart.org
Phone: (heart and stroke information) 1-800-AHA-USA1

Cardiac surgery patient information:
Website: www.heart-surgeon.com

The Society of Thoracic Surgeons:
Website: www.sts.org (look under "patient information")
Phone: 312-644-6610

Notes and Questions for the Doctor or Nurse:

Chapter Six

Diseases and Injury of the Brain and Spinal Cord

Head Injury

Another name for head injury is TBI (traumatic brain injury). Motor vehicle accidents cause the majority of these head injuries. Closed head injury means that the scalp and/or skull are intact enough so that the brain is not exposed to the environment outside, and open head injury means that the brain is exposed to the outside.

After an injury, swelling of the brain (cerebral edema) may occur, and as a result, pressure will increase in the skull. This increased intracranial pressure (ICP) can cause injury to the brain cells. In addition, blood clots may form and cause injury to the brain as well, and with the addition of severe brain swelling (edema), it may be impossible for the brain to overcome the pressure. At this point, the pressure can force the brain in the skull down onto the brainstem, causing a life-threatening event called herniation.

Head injuries will result in variable degrees of loss of consciousness, affecting the patient's ability to respond to the environment. This level of alertness may range from alert and mildly confused to coma. Coma is a complete loss of consciousness and inability to respond to the external environment, except with primitive reflexes.

33

Neurosurgeons often refer to "mass lesions" when discussing head injury patients. Most commonly, these are hematomas and contusions: when a blood clot is in the brain or on its surface it is called a hematoma; a contusion is basically a bruised brain. Hematomas that occur between the skull and the dura (thick membrane surrounding the brain) are called epidural hematomas. Subdural hematomas occur between the dura and the surface of the brain. Intracerebral hematomas are blood clots that are found within the brain tissue itself. Subarachnoid hemorrhage refers to diffuse blood that is spread thinly over the brain surface. In general, the hematomas and contusions described above are often seen on x-ray procedures such as CT (computerized tomography) scans. However, some traumatic brain injuries (TBI) can produce small changes that can't be seen on the CT scan but are scattered widely throughout the brain. These injuries are called "diffuse brain injuries." One type of diffuse brain injury is ischemia, which refers to inadequate blood supply to certain parts of the brain.

Skull Fractures

Most simple skull fractures require no treatment. Of greater concern is that the force causing the skull fracture may have damaged the brain itself. Basilar skull fractures are worrisome if they involve arteries, nerves, or other structures. Depressed skull fractures involve part of the bone pressing on the brain and may require surgical treatment. If a fracture extends into the sinuses, there may be a leak of CSF (cerebrospinal fluid) from the ears or nose. Although many of these leaks resolve by themselves, it may be necessary for the surgeon to place a lumbar drain (long thin tube inserted into the CSF space in the spine of the lower back). This relieves the pressure so that the leak in the base of the skull has time to heal.

Seizures From TBI

Seizures (fits or convulsions) may occur whenever brain injury occurs. Medical staff can give medications when the seizure occurs, but they may also give them before a seizure occurs, as a preventative measure.

Treatment of TBI

Certainly treatment of head injury depends on how severe the injury is. Many individuals with moderate or severe head injury undergo surgery in order to decrease the increased intracranial pressure (ICP) by removing blood clots or by releasing the pressure in obstructed brain ventricles (fluid spaces in the center of the brain). After surgery, the patient is taken back to the ICU for further monitoring and care. While in the ICU, the health care team will assist brain healing by maintaining the appropriate blood pressure and blood oxygen levels, and by monitoring brain pressure levels. Physicians use various devices that are designed to monitor changes in the patient's condition. Neurosurgeons can place an ICP monitor into the brain itself to detect excessive brain swelling (edema). One common ICP monitor is called a ventriculostomy. A ventriculostomy is a narrow, flexible hollow tube that is placed into the ventricles in the center of the brain in order to monitor ICP and also to drain CSF if the pressure increases. There are also other monitoring devices to assist the health care team in the goal of monitoring the head injury patient while in the intensive care unit.

Ruptured Cerebral Aneurysm & Subarachnoid Hemorrhage

An aneurysm is a bulging sac on one of the blood vessels that supplies the brain. This condition is common in adults, and can be associated with aging, high blood pressure, trauma, heredity, or diabetes. An aneurysm can rupture suddenly, even during sleep. This rupture can cause severe headaches, nausea and vomiting, sensitivity to light, neck pain and stiffness, memory loss, paralysis, and coma. The diagnosis can be made with a CT scan, which can show blood inside the skull, and an angiogram is used to find the source of the bleeding. While in the ICU, the patient is placed in a quiet, restful area in order to prevent the aneurysm from rupturing again. Oxygen is often given to the individual by mask or nasal prongs, and if necessary, a ventilator may be used to help the patient breathe and also to help control intracranial pressure when other measures fail. Medications are given as needed to relieve stress, control blood pressure and pain and also to maintain fluid balance.

Various monitoring devices are used in the ICU for patients with brain injuries. These include ICP monitors to monitor changes in intracranial pressure, pulmonary artery catheters to monitor heart pressures and fluid balance, arterial lines to measure changes in blood pressure, as well as the other usual ICU monitoring devices described in Chapter 1.

Surgery for ruptured cerebral aneurysms is done only when the patient's condition otherwise is good, and is performed mainly to relieve pressure on the brain from a blood clot, or to place a "clip" on the neck of the aneurysm in order to prevent another rupture. The blood vessels around the aneurysm will sometimes go into "spasm" (tightening and narrowing of blood vessels is called "vasospasm"). This vasospasm is monitored very closely, for prompt treatment is the goal of the ICU team.

Epilepsy

Epilepsy is a condition that occurs due to sudden brief changes in brain cell function, causing loss of consciousness and abnormal movements. These are called seizures. Generalized or tonic-clonic seizures occur when the whole brain is overloaded with electrical impulses. The person will fall to the ground unconscious, and then the body becomes stiff and jerking movements begin. Shallow breathing, or even brief moments of loss of breathing may occur. After a minute or two, the jerking movements slow down and the seizure stops. Bladder or bowel control may have been lost, and when the individual awakes, he or she will be sleepy and confused. Other types of seizures may also occur and may show up in different and often less dramatic ways.

Patients with seizures usually do not need to be in the ICU unless their seizures are continuous, repetitive and difficult to control with medications. Rarely, breathing may not resume when a seizure is over, and then the patient may need a ventilator to maintain breathing (see Chapter 3). This will cause the patient to be transferred to the ICU for further care.

Stroke (CVA)

When blood flow to a certain area of the brain is interrupted, a stroke occurs. This may happen when a blood clot blocks an artery or when the blood vessel breaks. Brain cells around the area of the stroke are destroyed for lack of blood, and this area of dead cells is called an infarct. After a stroke occurs, certain functions such as memory, body movements and speech may be lost. What is lost depends on the area of brain involved, as well as the size of the infarct. Patients with strokes are not always sent to the ICU for treatment unless they need the close monitoring that is available in the ICU.

For example, the patient may develop alterations in level of consciousness that affect breathing ability, and due to the difficulties these patients have with keeping their air passages clear, they can develop pneumonia. If they do, it may cause enough problems with breathing that ICU care is necessary. Abnormal blood pressure or heart rate patterns may also require treatment in the ICU.

Spinal Cord Injury

Approximately 450,000 people live with spinal cord injuries (SCI) in the U.S. Unfortunately, there are about 10,000 new cases per year, usually involving males age 16-30. Most commonly, these injuries happen in motor vehicle accidents, falls, and violence.

It is important to review at this time some basic anatomy before going on any further. The spinal cord is a large bundle of nerves that transmits electrical signals from the brain to the body. It is surrounded by rings of bone called vertebra. SCI occurs because of damage to the spinal cord, which then results in loss of function such as loss of feeling or ability to move an arm or leg. An important point here is that the higher in the spinal cord the injury occurs, the more complications or problems the patient will suffer.

The eight vertebrae in the neck are called "cervical" vertebrae; the top vertebra is called C1, the one below is called C2, etc. The "thoracic" vertebrae are the twelve vertebrae in the chest; the "lumbar" vertebrae are in the low back between the thoracic vertebrae and the pelvis, and the "sacral" vertebrae extend from the pelvis to the end of the spinal cord. Major nerves controlling muscle function and feeling come out from the spinal cord in between the vertebrae.

A complete injury to the spinal cord means there is no function below the level that is injured, while an incomplete injury means there is some remaining function below the level of injury.

Severe Cervical (neck) injuries usually result in quadriplegia (loss in function of arms and legs). In fact, injuries that occur above C4 in the neck will affect the patient's ability to breathe because of loss of diaphragm function. These patients will need a ventilator machine to maintain breathing.

Injuries at the thoracic level may result in paraplegia (leg paralysis) with the hands unaffected. Other effects from SCI include difficulty controlling body temperature, low blood pressure, chronic pain, inability to sweat below the level of injury, skin breakdown, and pulmonary emboli (see Chapter 4 for description of pulmonary emboli).

Patients with SCI's above thoracic level T4 are predisposed to problems with lung function due to loss of chest wall muscles. They may develop pneumonia, atelectasis, or aspiration of stomach contents (see chapter 4).

Obviously, patients with severe brain or spinal cord damage can be very ill and require careful, concentrated care while in the ICU. Depending on the situation, your loved one may require multiple procedures. These may include CT scans, MRI (magnetic resonance imaging) scans, EEG (electroencephalograph), central lines, "Swan-Ganz" catheters, ICP monitors, ventilators, intravenous medications, feeding tubes, and possibly surgery. Hopefully, after reading this chapter, you have a better understanding of why these procedures are necessary, and what crucial information they provide to the medical staff. Medical science is always changing, and new devices are always being invented to improve patient care.

Suggested Resources for Additional Information:

Heart and stroke information: American Heart Association
Website: www.americanheart.org
Stroke information: 1-888-4-stroke

National Stroke Association
9707 East Easterlane
Englewood, Co 80112
Website: www.stroke.org
Phone: 1-800-strokes

Epilepsy Foundation of America
4351 Garden City Drive
Landover, Maryland 20785
Phone: 1-800-332-1000

Notes and Questions for the Doctor or Nurse:

_____

_____

_____

_____

_____

_____

_____

_____

_____

_____

_____

_____

_____

_____

_____

_____

_____

_____

_____

_____

_____

_____

_____

_____

_____

_____

_____

Chapter Seven

Diseases of the Kidney

The main job of the kidneys is to filter waste products and excess fluids from the blood. One kidney is adequate doing this alone, but if both kidneys fail, a patient could die without medical intervention.

Kidney failure may be caused by diabetes, uncontrolled high blood pressure, kidney infections, kidney stones, gout, lupus, and many other illnesses. While some of these diseases cause a gradual loss of kidney function over the years (chronic renal failure), some illnesses cause the kidneys to stop working suddenly (acute renal failure).

A brief list of these illnesses include: severe overwhelming infection in the bloodstream (sepsis), trauma from accidents, and shock associated with sudden, severely low blood pressure from any cause.

Dialysis is a treatment method that takes over the "filtering" or "cleaning" function of the natural kidneys when they stop working properly. Hemodialysis is a process that filters blood from the body into a machine that cleans the blood of harmful waste products and then returns this blood to the body. Hemodialysis requires access to a large blood vessel. In the acute (sudden) situation, your physician will place a central line for access (see Chapter 2). If the need for dialysis becomes permanent, two surgical methods can give ready access to the bloodstream: An A-V fistula and a vascular graft. A fistula is created by surgically connecting a vein to a nearby artery, thus enlarging the vein for easier access with a needle. A graft is a manmade tube that is sewn between the vein and artery.

Peritoneal dialysis is a different dialysis cleansing technique that takes advantage of the peritoneal membrane that lines the abdominal cavity. With peritoneal dialysis, a soft, flexible catheter is placed into the abdominal cavity, and a special solution is then infused through the catheter into the abdomen for a few hours. After a few hours of "dwell time," this fluid is then allowed to drain out of the peritoneal cavity through the catheter. This drainage will also remove chemicals, fluid, and waste products, similar to the way hemodialysis removes them from the blood.

Patients who have chronic kidney failure may undergo kidney transplantation, depending on the situation. Like other organ transplants, patients with kidney transplants often go to the ICU after their surgery. These patients will be watched closely in the ICU, with special attention to fluid balance, vital functions, and observation for signs of infection. Kidney failure patients receive medications that prevent the body from "rejecting" the transplanted organ, and these important medications may also have a side effect of lowering immune system function, thus increasing the risk for developing various infections. Antibiotics are therefore also very important tools to combat these infections.

There are different conditions or diseases that can cause kidney failure, either temporary or permanent. Luckily, physicians today have the lifesaving tools and technology to diagnose and treat these conditions. After reading this chapter, I hope you will have a better understanding of why your loved one may need dialysis, what types of dialysis technology are available, and what types of procedures are necessary before dialysis can begin. This is a good knowledge base for additional important discussions with your physicians.

Suggested Resources for Additional Information:

National Kidney Foundation
30 East 33rd St.
NY, NY 10016
Website: www.kidney.org
Ph. 800-622-9010

Notes and Questions for the Doctor or Nurse:

Chapter Eight
Diseases of the Abdomen and Abdominal Surgery

The Acute Abdomen

Certain conditions that affect organs in the abdomen (large and small intestine, gall bladder, spleen etc.), whether from injury or underlying disease, may cause severe pain, fever and even shock (low blood pressure, sweating, fast heart rate and trouble breathing). These sudden emergencies involving the abdomen are called the "acute abdomen" because they often require emergency or urgent surgery, and may require a stay in the ICU either before or just after surgery. Depending on how severe the illness, your loved one may need the assistance of a ventilator after surgery (Chapter 3), and may require various monitoring devices as well while in the ICU. In addition to the usual heart rate, blood pressure, and oxygen monitoring devices, the patient may need to have a central or "CVP" line, arterial catheter, and "Swan-Ganz" catheter (see Chapter 2).

The peritoneum is a sac or membrane that surrounds the organs within the abdominal cavity. Many causes of acute abdominal disease involve peritonitis. Peritonitis is infection, irritation, or inflammation of the peritoneum. Peritonitis can be caused by a number of things including rupture of an organ such as the appendix, or obstruction or strangulation of the small bowel. Infection-causing bacteria get into the peritoneum either by rupture of an organ (like a stomach ulcer) or by escape through the diseased wall of an organ.

Abdominal injury from accidents or trauma may also cause shock from blood loss. Bleeding can occur from injured organs such as the liver or spleen, as well as from torn blood vessels. This bleeding requires surgical treatment, and often blood transfusions may be required (see Chapter 10). Hemorrhage may also occur from bleeding stomach ulcers or enlarged veins in the esophagus (varices). These conditions often require endoscopy (EGD) in order to make a diagnosis and assist with treatment. An EGD procedure involves putting a tube with optical capability down the mouth into the esophagus and stomach so that the physician can see the bleeding sites. Bleeding from varices can be treated in multiple ways, depending on the situation. This may include medications, endoscopic ligation or "banding" of the bleeding vessel, and injection of certain medicines into the bleeding vessel to stop the bleeding. The next section of this chapter describes specific abdominal diseases or conditions that require ICU care or surgery.

Pancreatitis

Acute or sudden pancreatitis occurs when digestive enzymes start to destroy the pancreas. Although this is not an infection, it starts a process of inflammation and release of toxic chemicals that is very similar to a severe infection. Acute pancreatitis is usually caused by either alcohol or stones in the gall bladder or bile duct. Signs of pancreatitis may include fever, fast heart rate, abdominal pain, elevated white blood cell count, and high levels of pancreatic enzymes in the blood. When pancreatitis is severe, it can cause problems with fluids, acid-base imbalance, electrolyte abnormalities, kidney failure, and ARDS (adult respiratory distress syndrome). (see Chapters 3,4,7,10). Physicians often treat pancreatitis by correcting and monitoring these complications, providing nasogastric or oralgastric suction and nutrition to "rest" the pancreas, such as TPN (total parenteral nutrition) or jejunal feedings (see Chapter 2).

Other complications that can occur in pancreatitis are infections and pancreatic pseudocysts. Pseudocysts are collections of pancreatic juice that are enclosed within a wall of tissue. When they become infected, they require drainage, either by placing a catheter through the skin into the pseudocyst, or directly by surgery.

Gall Bladder Disease

The majority of the cases of inflamed gall bladder come from gallstones that become impacted or lodged in the duct that empties the gall bladder, setting up an area of chemical inflammation that may eventually become infected. These areas may develop into abscesses or even gangrene of the gall bladder. Acute cholecystitis (gall bladder attack) usually causes the patient to experience fever, pain in the right upper part of the abdomen, elevated white blood count, and abnormalities on ultrasound or other x-ray tests. Initially, the patient will be treated with intravenous fluids, NG (nasogastric) suction, and antibiotics. For individuals in the ICU with severe disease or peritonitis (infection of the peritoneum), emergency surgery is necessary. There may also be other reasons that your physician will recommend surgery, however, this depends on the situation.

Perforated Duodenal Ulcer

Patients with this condition experience sudden pain in the middle of the upper abdomen that may travel to the right shoulder blade. Stomach contents are spilled into the abdomen from the ulcer hole in the duodenum and cause infection and peritionitis. Treatment may include fluids, antibiotics, nasogastric or orogastric suction, and surgery.

Small Bowel Obstruction

These patients have pain, vomiting, and "bloating" of the abdomen. Your physician may order plain x-rays of the abdomen (KUB), upper gastrointestinal (UGI) barium studies, barium enema, or CT scans in order to make the diagnosis, depending on its location and nature. Patients with small bowel obstruction have nasogastric or orogastric tubes placed into the stomach to remove gastric contents. If the obstruction is only partial, the individual may not need surgery. However, if the obstruction is complete, surgery will be necessary

Bowel Ischemia

Ischemia means inadequate blood supply to an organ. Bowel ischemia can be the result of occlusion of the arteries or veins supplying the bowel. Usually, a clot travels from another part of the body to the blood vessel that supplies the bowel, or a clot forms by itself in the bowel artery or vein. Sometimes bowel ischemia occurs in patients who are ill for other reasons such as major trauma, pancreatitis, heart attack, or the use of drugs that decrease blood flow in an artery that supplies the bowel. Individuals with bowel ischemia require intravenous fluids to maintain good blood pressure, and if they have peritonitis, surgery is required. If the patient doesn't have peritonitis, an angiogram test can be ordered if necessary. An angiogram is a procedure that injects dye through a catheter placed into an artery for x-rays to be made of the blood vessel. If the blood vessel is found to be completely occluded, the patient may be taken to the operating room to attempt to correct the problem. If the vessel is not completely occluded, other nonsurgical treatment options are available.

Large Bowel Obstruction

About 20% of patients with cancer of the colon or rectum also suffer from large bowel obstruction. Other causes include diverticulitis and volvulus. (diverticulitis is inflammation and leakage from a small colon "pouch" and volvulus is a twist or folding of the bowel). X-rays of various types can help make the diagnosis. Patients with complete obstruction or perforation of the bowel need intravenous fluids, antibiotics, and surgery. Your physician will consider other treatment options if there is only partial obstruction of the large bowel.

Abdominal Aortic Aneurysm

An aneurysm is a weak spot in the wall of a blood vessel that can "balloon out" and eventually break. In addition, bleeding can occur through a defect in the wall of the aorta (large artery in the abdomen). This is called aortic dissection. If the aneurysm leaks or blood loss occurs from the aortic dissection, the patient can develop shock and may need emergency surgery to repair the aorta.

Liver Failure

Failure of the liver can be acute (sudden), chronic, or fulminant (see next paragraph). Acute liver failure usually occurs in patients who suddenly develop hepatitis or liver injury from some cause, and these individuals don't have a history of liver disease. Typically, these patients have yellow eyes and skin (jaundice), easy bleeding, and very abnormal blood tests of liver function.

Encephalopathy refers to a patient with liver disease who becomes confused, disoriented, or excessively sleepy. Patients have fulminant liver failure if they develop encephalopathy within 8 weeks of the start of jaundice from their sudden liver injury. There are approximately 2,000 cases of fulminant liver failure in the U.S. per year. Fulminant liver failure is most often due to excess acetominophen, drug toxicity, hepatitis B and hepatitis A. Unfortunately, the cause of some cases cannot be found.

The treatment of fulminant liver failure in the ICU requires close monitoring for potential complications. For example, medicines are given to prevent bleeding in the gastrointestinal tract. These individuals may have a tendency to bleed excessively, since the injured liver no longer produces enough factors to clot blood properly.

Encephalopathy in chronic liver diseases is associated with too much ammonia in the blood. In order to reduce the level of blood ammonia, physicians may limit protein in the diet, provide lactulose, and give certain oral antibiotics. Unlike chronic liver failure, the encephalopathy found in acute liver disease is usually related to brain swelling (cerebral edema). Your physician will order medicines to reduce the brain swelling, and sometimes an ICP (intracranial pressure) monitor is necessary in order to measure brain pressure (see Chapter 6).

Liver transplantation is the only treatment that has been proven to improve survival in patients with fulminant liver failure and severe encephalopathy. The problem with transplantation at this time is the limited availability of organs for donation. At the end of 1998, there were more than 12,000 patients on the waiting list for liver transplants in the U.S.

There are many causes for the "acute abdomen." This chapter has provided a brief review of some of the more frequent causes as well as a description of how complications can occur, and what procedures may be necessary to diagnose and treat these abdominal illnesses.

Suggested Resources for Additional Information:

American College of Surgery
Website: www.facs.org
(look under "patient and public services")

American College of Gastroenterology
4900B South 31st Street Arlington, VA 22206
Phone: 703-820-7400
Website: www.acg.gi.org (look under "patient information")

Notes and Questions for the Doctor or Nurse:

Chapter Nine
Shock

S hock is a condition of the human body in which a severe abnormality has caused the circulatory system (heart, blood vessels, and oxygen supply) to fail to provide adequate support to organs and cells. Nearly all patients with shock from whatever cause have severely low blood pressure, fast heart rate and respiratory rate, diminished alertness, cold-clammy skin, decreased urine flow, and acid in the blood (low blood pH). Shock may be caused by heart failure (cardiogenic shock) because the heart is not pumping with enough force or "horsepower" to provide enough blood flow to vital organs and tissues. In addition, shock may also be caused by blood loss either from trauma or other causes. The decreased volume of blood in the body is the primary culprit in this situation. The final major cause of shock is severe infection (septic shock). In septic shock, a patient's temperature may be either high or low and the skin may be warm instead of cool and clammy as seen in other causes of shock. There is usually a site of infection that often infects the bloodstream. A blood test called the "white blood cell count" may be very high, or very low in severe infections. Other less common causes of shock may include severe dehydration without blood loss, failure of the adrenal glands, heat stroke, severe allergic reactions, and spinal cord injuries.

The treatment of shock depends upon the reason it occurred in the first place, however, in all cases, the medical team works hard to stabilize the patient's cardiovascular system (blood pressure and heart rate) as well as urine output. For example, in shock due to blood loss, physicians will order blood transfusions and intravenous fluids while they control the bleeding. In cardiogenic shock, medicines are given to allow the heart to pump with more vigor or "horsepower." In traumatic shock, injuries may require surgical repair and an IV will be necessary for blood transfusions and fluids. And finally, in septic shock, blood pressure is stabilized by giving fluids, pockets of infection are drained, and antibiotics are given according to the source and type of infection. No matter what the cause of shock, if blood pressure remains dangerously low despite fluids and other stabilizing treatments, strong intravenous medications called "pressors" may be necessary. Basically, pressors are drugs that constrict blood vessels and/or improve the pumping action of the heart in order to increase blood pressure.

In order to monitor these critically ill patients, various devices may need to be inserted into your loved one's blood vessels in order to provide important information about the progress of their treatment. For example, a pulmonary artery catheter may be needed in order to monitor heart pressures and blood output from the heart (cardiac output). The information that your physician obtains from this catheter will help him or her to decide how much fluid to give or what drugs to provide to resolve the shock (see Chapter 2). Another common device that may be placed is an arterial catheter ("art-line"). This device will continually monitor changes in blood pressure perhaps more accurately than a standard blood pressure arm cuff, and has the advantage of providing easy access for drawing arterial blood gases without separate needle sticks (see Chapter 2).

Not uncommonly, you will find that if your loved one is in shock from whatever cause, he or she may be placed on a ventilator machine (see Chapter 3) to support breathing while the vigorous process to restore blood pressure and kidney output continues. Once the shock improves significantly, the process of getting the patient off the ventilator can begin.

After reading this chapter, you should have a better understanding of just how complex shock is. This complexity clearly involves many organ systems, and requires multiple procedures and ICU resources for aggressive treatment. Researchers are working hard at finding safe, more effective treatments for shock. Hopefully, a new treatment for septic shock will be available in the near future.

Notes and Questions for the Doctor or Nurse:

Chapter Ten

Miscellaneous Diseases and Conditions

Endocrine Disorders

Endocrine disorders involve abnormalities of several organs including thyroid, pancreas, pituitary, and adrenal glands. Fortunately, with the exception of severe complications of diabetes, these disorders are relatively uncommon in the intensive care setting. Clearly, the most common endocrine disorder that results in ICU admission is diabetic ketoacidosis (DKA).

DKA occurs in diabetic patients when there is a complete or near complete absence of the hormone produced by the pancreas called insulin. Symptoms include fatigue, frequent urination, thirst, nausea, vomiting, and abdominal discomfort. The patient will frequently come in with difficulty breathing, diminished alertness or coma, low blood pressure, and significant dehydration. Patients commonly will have very high blood sugar levels, and also high levels of acids (keto-acids) in the bloodstream. This can be a very serious illness that requires prompt, aggressive treatment. This treatment includes insulin given by continuous infusion into a vein, intravenous fluids, and close monitoring of sodium and potassium (electrolyte) levels in the blood stream. These patients do not usually require a ventilator machine (see Chapter 3); however, this may be necessary in a patient who is severely ill.

Electrolyte Disorders

Electrolytes refer to blood levels of certain essential salts or minerals that can be measured in the blood stream. The most common examples include sodium, potassium, calcium, and magnesium. When these salts and minerals in the bloodstream become imbalanced, the body can have problems which vary depending on the severity of the imbalance.

Disorders of sodium balance can occur when there is either too much sodium or too little sodium in the bloodstream. Low blood sodium can occur from many causes, however it most commonly results as a side effect from use of water pills (diuretics), vomiting, diarrhea, heart failure, cirrhosis of the liver or kidney failure. Depending on the cause, patients may be dehydrated, have normal body fluid status, or even have too much fluid "on board." Therefore, treatment may include either giving intravenous salt solutions (saline), or restricting fluid intake, depending on the individual situation.

Too much sodium in the blood usually occurs when more water is lost from the body than salt. This most commonly will occur with vomiting, diarrhea, severe sweating, high blood sugar levels, and certain medications. These patients are usually very ill, and oftentimes are confused or sleepy as a side effect from the high sodium levels. Therapy usually will include giving water and other solutions directly into a vein.

High calcium levels can result from several different causes and symptoms may include constipation, decreased appetite, abdominal pain, weakness, sleepiness, and even coma. Treatment options include giving salt solutions directly into a vein, and various medications. Dialysis (see Chapter 7) may be necessary for severely increased calcium levels.

Low calcium levels also occur from multiple causes, and symptoms may include muscle spasms, tingling around the mouth/lips, low heart rate and blood pressure, and even seizures. Therapy may include giving the patient either oral or intravenous calcium supplements. Whether the patient receives oral or intravenous supplements depends on how low the levels are, and whether the patient is having those symptoms.

High magnesium levels occur most often in patients with kidney disease, or in patients who are receiving magnesium-containing medications. Patients with high magnesium levels may experience weakness; at even higher levels individuals may develop trouble breathing or low heart rate and blood pressure. Treatment includes withdrawing certain medications and giving other medications to help correct the problem, as well as dialysis for patients with kidney failure.

Low magnesium levels are fairly common in the ICU, and the usual reason is that the mineral is lost from the gastrointestinal tract or from the kidney. For example, this may occur after severe diarrhea or vomiting, as well as from diuretic medications.

High potassium levels will result from many conditions, however it is particularly common in patients with kidney disease who take potassium-containing medications. Your physician will be concerned about the effects very high potassium levels may have on the heart rhythm, and multiple medications are available to reverse this problem.

Low potassium levels may are also a cause for concern, and treatment may include oral as well as intravenous potassium replacement. It is not uncommon to find low magnesium levels together with low potassium levels.

Bleeding Disorders

Of all the patients in ICUs, 40% experience bleeding of some type. However, severe bleeding is relatively rare. This section will give more detail on a few of the disorders that cause bleeding.

DIC

DIC (disseminated intravascular coagulation) occurs when clotting and then unclotting occurs throughout the blood stream.

The result is that some products in the blood that help with clotting (platelets and clotting factors) become used up or consumed. This loss of clotting factors causes the patient to have an abnormal tendency to bleed. Some of the common causes of this abnormal bleeding tendency include shock (of any cause), severe infection (sepsis), traumatic injuries, problems with childbirth, transfusion reactions and others. DIC can be difficult to diagnose at times, and treatment may include transfusion of certain blood products and factors, as well as treatment of the disease that caused it in the first place.

Liver Failure

Liver failure may cause bleeding as well and may require transfusion with platelets and other blood products. Alcoholic cirrhosis, viral hepatitis, septic shock, and other conditions can cause liver failure (see Chapter 8).

Low Platelet Counts

Low levels of platelets in the blood may cause bleeding, as well as affecting how well the platelets themselves work. TTP (thrombotic thrombocytopenic purpura) and ITP (idiopathic thrombocytopenic purpura) are diseases that cause low platelet counts, and the treatment options in these relatively rare diseases are different between the two diseases. Other causes of low platelets include DIC (disseminated intravascular coagulation), bone marrow cancers, some infections, and side effects from certain medications. If the levels of platelets become severely reduced, or significant bleeding occurs from the low platelet levels, transfusions of platelets can be given.

Bleeding Due To Medications

Often medications are given in order to prevent blood clots from forming in blood vessels, or to destroy blood clots that have already formed. Since these medications will interfere with blood clotting, individuals may be more likely to bleed after taking these medications. Your physician will monitor the situation and treatment is readily available to reverse this bleeding tendency if it becomes a problem.

Blood Transfusions

It may become necessary for your physician to order a blood transfusion for your family member or loved one. There are several different blood products available, depending on the specific need of the individual. The most common choices of transfusion products for your physician to consider include whole blood, packed red blood cells, plasma, plasma factors, and platelets. Packed red blood cells may be given when severe anemia or blood loss occurs together with evidence of low levels of blood oxygen. Low levels of blood oxygen from severe anemia can cause angina (heart chest pain), confusion and fainting, heart failure and heart rhythm problems. Platelets are transfused when platelets in the blood are very low, or when they are too low for the patient to tolerate a surgical procedure. Fresh frozen plasma is given to replace certain blood factors. In addition, plasma is used to reverse the "blood-thinning" effects of the drug "Coumadin" (a trade name for warfarin) when the bleeding tendency is severe.

Cross Matching And Transfusion Reactions

Red blood cells from donor and recipient patients are matched by combining these cells at 2 different temperatures (cross-matching). This takes time, but is very important to do in order to avoid transfusion reactions. Cross matching is therefore more than just matching for standard ABO blood type.

Significant transfusion reactions can occur from the transfusion of mismatched or incompatible blood. This may cause destruction of the transfused red cells and release of harmful toxins into the blood stream. Severe reactions may cause low blood pressure, kidney problems, DIC (disseminated intravascular coagulation), and ARDS (adult respiratory distress syndrome) (see Chapter 4). The medical team is trained to recognize this rare problem promptly, and when recognized, the team will stop the transfusion and begin treatment. Fever is a less severe reaction that can occur after some transfusions and is usually treated with medicines to lower the temperature. Hives can occur also, and these reactions are usually treated with antihistamine drugs.

Risks of Disease Transmission from Blood Transfusions

The chances of developing hepatitis from blood transfusions are few. All blood is tested for hepatitis B, and the current screening test for hepatitis C detects 90% of infected blood. Post transfusion hepatitis occurs in 1 out of every 63,000 transfusions.

The risk of AIDS is less than 1 per 493,000 transfusions.

CMV (cytomegalovirus) transmission can occur in 3 to 12 patients per 100 units of blood transfused. CMV infection causes an infection similar to mononucleosis, and also causes disease of the eye (retina) in AIDS patients, as well as pneumonia in other patients who have poor immune systems. The highest risk individuals are bone marrow recipients who do not have antibodies to CMV who receive marrow from a donor who has been infected in the past. Other patients vulnerable to CMV include premature or low birth-weight infants, cancer and AIDS patients as well as those who have had their spleens removed. It is not usually a problem in patients without these risks.

Although precautions and testing generally prevent complications from transfusions, there still may be ill effects. It is important to discuss this with your physician.

Alternatives To The Use Of Blood Bank Products

Most blood banks will allow anyone who is planning to have surgery to donate his/her blood 2 to 3 weeks before their surgery (autologous donation). The patient will need to take iron or erythropoietin after donating blood and prior to surgery. Sometimes family members want to designate members of their immediate family as possible donors of blood, if needed, with the idea that family members are less likely to have infectious diseases that can be transmitted. Interestingly, the medical information available shows that in comparison to regular volunteer donors who have been screened, designated donor blood is more likely to test positive for infectious diseases and therefore is not necessarily safer than volunteer donor blood from the blood bank.

Orthopedic Injuries

Patients with orthopedic injuries are those who have bone fractures, dislocations, joint and tendon injuries, etc. These patients do not usually require admission to the ICU. Unfortunately, patients who are in motor vehicle accidents or have suffered trauma from other causes may have multiple bone fractures as well as internal organ injuries. These patients with "multiple trauma" will most likely require intensive ICU care. This may include a ventilator, central lines, "Swan-Ganz" catheters and other technologies previously described in this text. Obviously, these patients will require the expertise of several surgical specialists, including perhaps bone (orthopedic), abdominal, chest (thoracic) and brain (neurosurgery).

Traumatic long-bone fractures themselves will require surgical treatment, however, complications may still occur. Fat embolism occurs when fat enters the bloodstream, causing trouble breathing, spotty bruising or "petechiae" in the skin, and mental confusion. This problem occurs most commonly after traumatic fracture to long bones, but also can occur when other fatty tissues are injured, such as the liver. The occurrence of fat embolism is unpredictable, and the treatment may require placing the patient temporarily on a ventilator until improvement occurs.

Individuals who have sustained significant blunt force injury may suffer a fracture of the pelvis. A small minority of these may become unstable with low blood pressure due to internal bleeding from the fracture. These patients will require intravenous fluids and perhaps blood transfusions in the ICU. In addition, the orthopedic surgeon will stabilize the fracture and provide appropriate treatment.

Pulmonary embolism may also occur (see Chapter 4) after long-bone fracture and pelvic fractures, but again, the incidence is variable and unpredictable. Physicians are aware of this possible complication, and may prescribe "blood-thinning" medications.

Bleeding abnormalities, anemia, blood transfusions, blood sugar problems, as well as disorders of salt and mineral balance are common in patients in the ICU. Since these disorders can cause complications, it isn't surprising that your loved one may have to have frequent blood tests to keep a close watch on these important blood values. In addition, bone fractures do not always require ICU care, but treatment in the ICU may become necessary when complications occur or multiple organs are injured.

Suggested Resources for Additional Information:

Diabetes: American Diabetes Association
National Office: 1701 North Beauregard St.
Alexandria, VA. 22311
Website: www.diabetes.org
Phone: 1-800-342-2383

Orthopedics: "Orthosearch"
Website: www.orthosearch.com
Look under "patient information"

Notes and Questions for the Doctor or Nurse:

Chapter Eleven
The Living Will
and Organ Donation

M ost of us don't like to think about things like illness and death. Unfortunately, each of us may face choices some-day about life and death issues. This chapter will attempt to assist you as a family member or friend of a critically ill patient as you try to deal with some of these difficult issues.

Medical science has advanced over the years to the point that many diseases can be treated successfully, often relying on sophisticated technology and advanced procedures. Sometimes this may mean that life-saving procedures are being provided for your loved one while you are unsure what his or her choice would have been if he or she were able to communicate. You see, most of us are able to make our own decisions; however, when severely ill in the ICU, patients may not be able to communicate these wishes to their family and health care staff.

End of life issues gained national attention back in 1975 with the case of Karen Ann Quinlan. Ms. Quinlan unfortunately suf-fered a respiratory arrest (stopped breathing) resulting in a coma; she was unable to breathe without a ventilator and unable to eat or drink. Her parents endured a long legal battle to get control of their daughter's fate. They argued that Karen would not have wanted to be kept alive with no hope of recovery. Eventually, the courts gave them the right to remove her from the ventilator machine, and she died several years later.

The debate over right-to-die issues has continued after the Quinlan case. After the U.S. Supreme Court affirmed a patient's right to control his/her own medical treatment in 1990, congress passed the Patient Self-Determination Act (PSDA) in 1991. Basically, this law gives all legally competent adults the right to make decisions today about the limits of health care treatment they would want to receive in the future if they became unable to communicate their wishes themselves. In addition, this law requires that all hospitals, nursing homes, and other health care facilities give all patients information about their right to have a legal document called an advance directive.

Advance Directives

An advance directive is a legal paper that tells doctors and other health care professionals how you would want medical decisions made if a future crisis would occur, even if you can't communicate these decisions for yourself. If you have this paper in your medical record, your doctors will be able to take care of you based on your wishes written in the advance directive. There are two kinds of advance directives. A **durable power of attorney for health care** decisions or a **health care proxy** allows you to specify someone such as a husband, wife, daughter, son, or close friend to act on your behalf if you are not able to make decisions for yourself. It is important that you ask this person if he or she is willing to act as your "agent." In addition, you should make sure this person knows what your short term and long term goals and values are with regard to your health care. If you don't have a durable power of attorney document, there may be confusion about who has authority to make end-of-life health care decisions for you. It is a misconception that these decisions about medical care can be automatically turned over to a spouse or close family member. Not all states have laws authorizing decision- making in the absence of advance directives.

A **living will** is the most common advance directive. It tells your doctor in writing what type of medical care you want or do not want if you should become unable to make the decisions yourself. Living wills can't possibly address every technological possibility in health care. It will usually focus on whether ventilators and artificial nutrition are acceptable, and under what circumstances they are allowed: temporary or long term. Several types of decisions can be made in a living will. The patient can choose to accept all the treatments recommended by the physician, accept some treatments and refuse others, or refuse all treatments.

CPR (cardiopulmonary resuscitation) is an emergency procedure used to revive a dying person whose heart has stopped. This includes external heart massage with chest compressions, electric shocks, drugs, and ventilators. CPR is one of the more common treatments that are included in advance directives. Other treatments that can be included in a living will are mechanical ventilation (Chapter 3), antibiotics, kidney dialysis (Chapter 7), blood transfusions (Chapter 10), and surgery.

The law in some states requires that there be certain conditions met before an advance directive can be honored. In addition, in some states certain treatments or procedures, once put in place, can't be stopped by an advance directive. You may want to consider talking to a lawyer in your state to see what treatments cannot be stopped once started. It is not a legal necessity, however, to have an attorney prepare the living will.

Choice in Dying, a national nonprofit organization dedicated to improving communication about end-of-life decisions, operates a website that includes each state's advance directive, along with instructions on how to complete one. Those individuals who have either told their physicians they don't want CPR (cardiopulmonary resuscitation) or a ventilator if they should either stop breathing or have a cardiac arrest, or have written this in an advance directive are referred to as "No Code" or DNR (do not resuscitate) on the hospital chart. It is important to note that this does not mean that all treatments are withheld, or that the staff will no longer provide care, it just means that CPR and ventilators will not be used on the patient. For example, if a "Code Blue" or "Code" is called in the hospital, emergency personnel will rush to the patient's bedside to attempt to resuscitate a patient who suffered a cardiac arrest (heart and breathing has stopped). However, if a DNR order is written on the chart, a "Code Blue" will not be called.

Organ Donation

The topic of organ donation is one that physicians and nurses hope to avoid as they work hard to save lives in the ICU. It is important for families to have accurate information about organ donation so that they can make informed decisions. Every year, thousands of people are given another chance in life by receiving an organ transplant. These life-saving transplants would not be possible without the generosity of organ donors and families who decide to donate the organs of their loved ones. For example, a blind person can see again with a cornea transplant; a patient with severe heart failure can live a healthier life with a heart transplant; and a patient with severe lung disease can breathe again after a lung transplant.

Clearly, patients benefit from organ donation, but families can also receive some benefit during their time of grieving. It is important for families to understand that something positive can come from a tragic situation. There is a great need for donated organs. Every day nearly 8 people die because not enough donated organs are available for those who desperately need them. Every 18 minutes, another child or adult is added to the waiting list for organ transplants in the United States.

The most important thing to do is to discuss organ donation with your family before the question occurs unexpectedly. Individuals who wish to donate their organs should sign a donor card or indicate his/her preference on their automobile driver's license. However, even if the patient has signed a donor card or indicated their preference on a driver's license, the family will be asked to sign a consent form before donation can begin. The question of organ donation may be brought up when the patient is on life support machines (ventilator) and further treatment is felt to be futile with little or no hope of a happy outcome.

Quite a few organs and tissues can be donated. For example, an organ donor can donate lungs, heart, kidneys, liver, intestine, and/or pancreas. Tissue donors can donate corneas, skin, heart valves, and bone. There are usually no age limits on who can donate. The main factor to be considered is the patient's condition. For example, the following conditions will eliminate the possibility of donation: diabetes, encephalitis, active severe infection (sepsis), cancer other than primary brain tumor, any transmittable disease, and death of unknown cause.

Each patient waiting for a transplant is listed with UNOS (United Network for Organ Sharing). This agency is responsible for making sure that organs are distributed fairly and equally. When a donor is found, the blood type of the donor, as well as tissue type, body weight and size, are matched against a list of patients who are waiting for a transplant. The severity of the recipient's illness and elapsed time on the waiting list are also factored into the matching process.

Finally, families should be reassured that there are no additional fees for organ donation, and highly skilled transplant surgeons make sure that the body will not be altered or disfigured, so that normal funeral arrangements can be carried out, including viewing of the body.

Advance directives, living wills and organ donation are subjects that certainly can be difficult to discuss not only for families, but for physicians as well. Physicians are trained to devote their energy primarily to saving lives, and they may find it difficult to withdraw procedures or remove life support from patients. Unfortunately, there are times when continued aggressive life support and complex procedures are not appropriate, and are actually futile. It is important that patients and families have discussions about advance directives and organ donation, if possible, before critical illness occurs.

Suggested Resources for Additional Information:

Choice in Dying
National Office
1035 30th St.
Washington, D.C. 20007
Website: www.choices.com
Phone: 1-800-989-WILL (9455)
This organization will provide you with specific living will documents for each Individual state, as well as further educational information about advance-directives.

ORGAN DONATION:
Coalition on Donation: 1-800-355-share
The purpose of this nonprofit alliance is to increase public awareness of organ and tissue donation, correct misconceptions about donation, and increase willingness to donate.

United Network for Organ Sharing (UNOS):
1-888-TX-INFO1
This nonprofit organization operates the Organ Procurement and Transplantation Network, and develops the national system to assure equal access for all patients needing organs for transplantation.

Glossary and Index

ABDOMINAL AORTIC ANEURYSM: (AAA or "Triple A") an abnormal bulging sac on the largest artery in the abdomen (Chapter 8).

ABG (arterial blood gas): a blood sample is drawn from a wrist artery, or art line (unlike the usual blood sample from a vein), and oxygen (O_2), carbon dioxide (CO_2) and pH (acid-base status) is measured (Chapter 3).

ACID-BASE IMBALANCE: this occurs when the normal pH of the blood becomes abnormal, causing the blood to have either too much acid or too much alkali or base (Chapter 8).

ACUTE PANCREATITIS: a condition that occurs when digestive enzymes suddenly start to attack the pancreas (Chapter 8).

ADRENAL GLANDS: a small gland that sits on top of each kidney. Cortisol is an important steroid hormone produced by this gland (Chapter 9).

ALLERGIC REACTIONS: severe allergic reactions may result most commonly from bee or insect stings and certain foods. This may result in hives, trouble breathing, and shock (Chapter 9).

ALPHA-1-ANTITRYPSIN DEFICIENCY: a hereditary type of emphysema caused by a deficiency of a certain protein. This causes disease at an early age (Chapter 4).

ALS (amyotrophic lateral sclerosis): a fatal disease of the nervous system that involves progressive paralysis of the muscles (Chapter 3).

AMMONIA: a compound that increases in the blood, usually due to liver disease (Chapter 8).

ANEURYSM: ("AN-your-ism") a weak spot in the wall of a blood vessel (artery) that can "balloon-out" and eventually break (Chapters 6 and 8).

ANGIOGRAM: ("AN-jeeo-gram") a long thin tube called a catheter is placed inside an artery in the groin or arm using local anesthesia. X-ray contrast fluid is then injected through the catheter and plaques or blockages in the artery can then be seen using x-ray equipment. Although this technique can be used to look at blood vessels in many organs, the most commonly known angiogram is called the cardiac catheterization. This procedure produces images of the coronary arteries that supply the heart (Chapters 5, 6).

ANGINA: ("AN-ji-nah"or "an JI-nah") a painful or uncomfortable feeling in the chest, back, arm, neck, or jaw. It is a warning that the heart muscle is not getting enough oxygen-rich blood. (Chapter 5).

ANGIOPLASTY (PTCA): ("AN-jeeo-plasty") a medical procedure that uses an inflatable balloon catheter to open a blocked coronary artery. This procedure may also be used on other blocked arteries, such as the legs (Chapter 5).

ANEMIA: hemoglobin is a molecule in the blood that carries oxygen. When hemoglobin values are low, it is called anemia. Anemia can be caused by blood loss as well as chronic diseases (Chapter 10).

AORTIC DISSECTION: ("dye-sek-shun") blood leaks into a defective area in the wall of the aorta (major artery that leaves the heart). The result is a bulging mass that may extend down the aorta and cause complications (Chapter 5).

APNEA OR SLEEP APNEA: refers to multiple episodes of "non-breathing" during sleep. This is associated with snoring, low oxygen levels, and daytime sleepiness (Chapter 4).

ARDS: (Adult Respiratory Distress Syndrome) in this condition, the lung becomes severely "injured," and fluid accumulation causes low oxygen levels and "stiff" lungs that require the ventilator for support (Chapter 4).

ART LINE (arterial catheter): a soft flexible catheter placed most commonly into a wrist artery using local anesthesia. Blood pressure can then be monitored continuously on a bedside monitor without using a blood pressure cuff. Blood samples to test for blood gas levels can also be drawn through this catheter easily and painlessly (Chapters 1, 8, and 9).

ATELECTASIS: ("Ata-Lek-tussis") a condition whereby a portion of the lung such as a lobe or segment, or even the whole lung itself may collapse (Chapter 4).

ATHERECTOMY: ("A-thur-EK-ta-mee") a procedure that uses a catheter and special cutting and grinding tools to remove plaque from the walls of coronary arteries (Chapter 5).

ATRIAL FIBRILLATION: a chaotic beating of the atrium of the heart that can be treated either with drugs or electric shock, depending on the specific situation (Chapter 5).

BASILAR SKULL FRACTURE: a fracture of the base of the skull. These patients may have bruises behind the ear or "Raccoon Eyes" (Chapter 6).

BLOOD PRESSURE: a common vital sign that is measured with a blood pressure cuff on the arm, or by placing an arterial catheter (art line) (Chapter 1).

BLOOD VESSELS: structures that carry blood (arteries, veins, capillaries and venules) (Chapter 8).

BIOPSIES: a piece of tissue is removed from an organ and examined in the lab (Chapter 4).

BOWEL ISCHEMIA: refers to poor blood supply to the bowel because of narrowing of the arteries that supply the bowel (Chapter 8).

BRADYCARDIA: (BRAY-dee-CAR-dee-a) a slow heart rate.

BRONCHODILATORS: ("Bron-ko-Dye-lay-tors") medicines that are given either by inhaled, oral, or intravenous routes to "open-up" or dilate breathing passages that are narrowed from spasm. They are commonly used in diseases such as asthma and COPD (Chapter 4).

BRONCHOSCOPY: ("bron-Kosk-up-pee") a type of endoscope (flexible tube with optical capabilities) that can be inserted under local anesthesia and sedation through the mouth, nose, endotracheal tube or tracheostomy. Doctors can use this scope to see all of the breathing passages of the lungs and take samples for biopsy and cultures, and remove mucous plugs (Chapter 4).

CABG: (coronary artery bypass surgery) the process of surgically bypassing blocked coronary arteries (Chapter 5).

CALCIUM: a mineral needed by the body that can be measured by a blood test (Chapter 10).

CARBON DIOXIDE OR CO2 LEVEL: the amount of carbon dioxide found in the blood. This measurement is made by drawing an arterial blood gas sample (ABG). (Chapter 3).

CARDIAC ARREST: an emergency in which the heart stops, or a severe electrical disturbance in heart rhythm causes blood circulation to cease. Emergency resuscitation may include CPR, mechanical ventilation, electrical therapy, and emergency medications (Chapter 11).

CARDIAC CATHETERIZATION: see Angiogram.

CARDIAC OUTPUT: refers to a measurement of blood flow out of the heart. This can be considered the "horsepower" or pumping power of the heart (Chapter 9).

CARDIOGENIC SHOCK: ("Kar-dee-o-JEN-ik") shock that is due to severe heart failure. In this condition, the heart is still beating, however the pumping action of the heart is much weaker than normal (Chapter 9).

CARDIOLOGIST: a physician who specializes in the diagnosis and non-surgical treatment of diseases of the heart (Chapter 5).

CARDIOMYOPATHY: a disease of the heart muscle of unknown cause (Chapter 5).

CARDIOTHORACIC SURGEON: a surgeon who specializes in the surgical treatment of heart and lung diseases (Chapter 5).

CARDIOVASCULAR: pertains to the heart and blood vessels (Chapters 5 and 9).

CATHETER: a soft, hollow, flexible tube that can be placed into blood vessels or body cavities (Chapter 7).

CCU: cardiac intensive care unit (preface).

CENTRAL LINE: a small soft tube (catheter) is temporarily inserted under local anesthesia into a large vein in the neck (internal jugular line) or under the collarbone (subclavian line) (Chapter 2).

CEREBRAL ANEURYSM: ("se-REE-brul AN-your-ism") a bulging sac on one of the arteries that supply the brain (Chapter 6).

CEREBRAL EDEMA: ("se-REE-brul eh-DEE-ma") swelling of the brain (Chapter 6).

CHEST TUBE: a tube, which is placed into the pleural cavity to drain off fluids and infections. In addition, a chest tube can drain air from a pneumothorax. These procedures are done under local anesthesia with sedatives (Chapter 4).

CHF: see congestive heart failure.

CHOLECYSTITIS: sudden gall bladder attack (Chapter 8).

CLOSED HEAD INJURY: a type of head injury where the brain is not exposed to the environment outside (Chapter 6).

COLON: refers to the large bowel or intestine (Chapter 8).

COLONOSCOPY: a long thin scope with optical capability (endoscope) is placed under local anesthesia into the colon to diagnose and treat disease.

COMA: complete loss of consciousness and the inability to respond to the external environment with anything other than primitive reflexes (Chapter 6).

CONGESTIVE HEART FAILURE: (CHF) a condition whereby the heart muscle pumps with less force and the heart chambers stretch and enlarge to hold more blood (Chapter 5).

COPD: (chronic obstructive pulmonary disease) includes diseases that are characterized by obstruction to airflow when breathing out, resulting in wheezing and trouble breathing. Typical diseases are: emphysema, chronic bronchitis, bronchiectasis, and asthma (Chapter 4).

CORONARY STENT: a device placed inside a coronary artery to keep it open after angioplasty (Chapter 5).

CPAP: ("see-pap") (continuous positive airway pressure) this refers to a ventilator machine that is set to provide continuous air pressure and oxygen, but not force breaths into the patient's lungs. This mode of ventilation is sometimes used when a patient is being "weaned" from the ventilator. CPAP may also be provided by a small portable machine that provides continuous air pressure through a mask that is placed over the nose or face. This (mask) mode of therapy is often used in patients with sleep apnea (Chapter 3).

CPR: (cardiopulmonary resuscitation) when a patient's heart stops beating and /or lungs stop breathing, trained personnel provide chest compressions and artificial breathing in an attempt to revive the patient. Non-medical people who learn the procedure from a course can also provide CPR (Chapter 11).

CSF: (cerebrospinal fluid) fluid that is normally found in chambers within the brain, and also surrounding the brain and spinal cord (Chapter 6).

CT ("CAT") SCAN: a complex x-ray imaging technique that helps to indirectly visualize internal organs in more detail than standard x-rays (Chapter 6).

CVA: (stroke or cerebrovascular accident) occurs when blood flow to a certain area of the brain is interrupted, killing or damaging brain cells (Chapter 6).

CVP LINE: (see CENTRAL LINE) a special intravenous catheter that is specifically used to measure pressures in the large veins emptying into the right atrium of the heart (Chapter 2).

CYSTIC FIBROSIS: a genetic disease characterized by airflow obstruction, progressive breathlessness, abnormalities of the pancreas, and recurrent infections (Chapter 4).

DEHYDRATION: a condition that occurs when the body loses more water than is replaced (chapter 10).

DEPRESSED SKULL FRACTURE: a fracture of the skull bone that presses on the brain (Chapter 6).

DIALYSIS: (hemodialysis) a process that filters blood from the body into a machine that cleans the blood of harmful waste products and returns the filtered blood back to the body. This process requires access to a large blood vessel (Chapter 7).

DIC: (disseminated intravascular coagulation) this condition occurs when "clotting" and then "unclotting" occurs throughout the bloodstream. This process results in spontaneous bleeding, and can occur as a result of shock (Chapter 10).

DIFFUSE BRAIN INJURY: an injury to the brain that produces multiple small changes that can't be seen on CT scan that are scattered widely throughout the brain (Chapter 6).

DIGESTIVE ENZYMES: proteins that are produced by the body to break down foods (Chapter 8).

DIVERTICULITIS: ("DI-ver-tick-U-light-us") an "outpouching"from the bowel wall that can become infected (Chapter 8).

DKA: (diabetic ketoacidosis) a condition of poorly controlled diabetes associated with high blood sugar levels, acid in the blood, dehydration, and electrolyte abnormalities (Chapter 10).

DNR: ("do not resuscitate") this order is written in the patient's chart, per advance directive, that no CPR or mechanical ventilation will be provided to the patient should cardiac arrest occur (Chapter 11).

DURA: the thick membrane that surrounds the brain (Chapter 6).

ECHOCARDIOGRAM: an ultrasound machine that provides an image of the heart and its chambers and valves (Chapter 5).

EEG: (electroencephalograph or "ee-Lek-troh-en-SEF-a-loh-graff") a procedure that monitors and records electrical brain wave activity by placing electrodes on the scalp and recording electrical activity. This does not provide a "shock" to the patient, and is painless (Chapter 6).

EGD: a long flexible tube with optical capabilities is placed into the mouth, down the esophagus (swallowing tube) into the stomach in order to diagnose and treat some gastrointestinal disorders. This procedure is done under local anesthesia and sedation (Chapter 8).

EKG: a paper tracing that shows the rhythm and characteristics of the electrical system of the heart (Chapter 5).

ELECTROLYTES: ("lytes") refers to a common blood test that analyzes levels of certain important salts and minerals such as Sodium, Potassium, Calcium etc. (Chapter 10).

EMPHYSEMA: ("em-fi-SEE-ma") a lung disease characterized by destruction of air sacs (alveoli) and lung tissue, progressive breathing trouble, and obstruction to airflow when exhaling (Chapter 4).

EMPYEMA: ("em-pie-EE-ma") infected, thick, acidic pleural effusion (Chapter 4).

ENCEPHALOPATHY: ("en-sef-a-Lop-a-thee") a disturbance in brain function from many causes, which varies from confusion to deep coma (Chapter 6).

ENDOCRINE: having to do with organs and glands such as the pituitary, pancreas, thyroid, and adrenal (Chapter 10).

ENDOCRINOLOGIST: a physician who has received specialized training in the diagnosis and non-surgical treatment of endocrine diseases (diabetes, thyroid, pituitary, etc.).

ENDOSCOPE: a flexible tube with optical capabilities.

ENDOSCOPY: ("en-DOS-kuppy") see EGD.

ENDOSCOPIC LIGATION OR BANDING: bleeding esophagus veins (varices) are treated by placing a band around the vein by using an endoscope (Chapter 8).

ENDOTRACHEAL ("en-doe-TRAY-kee-el") TUBE or (ET-TUBE): a hollow tube that is placed in the mouth or through the nostril into the trachea (windpipe) to provide direct access to the lungs. This tube is necessary to provide mechanical ventilation. (Chapter 3).

EPIDURAL HEMATOMA: a blood clot that is located between the skull and the dura (Chapter 6).

ENTERAL: a reference to feeding the patient by mouth or feeding tube directly into the stomach instead of using IV feeding (Chapter 2).

ESOPHAGEAL VARICES: an enlarged and tortuous vein in the esophagus that can bleed (Chapter 8).

EXTREMITY: arm or leg.

EXTUBATION OR EXTUBATE ("EX-too-BATE"): the act of removing the endotracheal tube when the patient no longer needs the ventilator (Chapter 3).

FULMINANT LIVER FAILURE: liver failure that is associated with encephalopathy within eight weeks of either liver injury or the start of jaundice (Chapter 8).

GALLBLADDER: a pear shaped organ located underneath the liver that holds bile (Chapter 8).

GALLSTONE: a solid object usually made of cholesterol that is produced and found in the gallbladder (Chapter 8).

GASTROENTEROLOGIST: a physician who specializes in the diagnosis and non-surgical treatment of diseases of the digestive tract.

GI: (gastrointestinal) refers to the esophagus, stomach, intestines, pancreas, and liver (Chapter 8).

G-TUBE: (gastrostomy tube) a feeding tube that is placed by a surgical incision on the skin, that then allows the tube to be anchored into the stomach (Chapter 2).

HEART RATE: a common vital sign that shows how fast the heart is beating (Chapter 1).

HEART RHYTHM: an indication of whether the heart rate or pulse rate is regular (no skipped beats) or irregular (skipped beats) (Chapter 1).

HEAT STROKE: a severe illness that occurs due to hot/humid exposure. Symptoms may include coma, bizarre behavior, hot flushed skin, fever, and low blood pressure (Chapter 9).

HEMATOLOGIST/ONCOLOGIST: a physician who specializes in the diagnosis and treatment of blood diseases and cancer.

HEMATOMA ("HE-ma-TOE-ma"): a blood clot (Chapter 6).

HEMODIALYSIS: see DIALYSIS.

HEMORRHAGE: refers to severe bleeding (Chapter 8).

HEMORRHAGIC SHOCK: see SHOCK: shock caused by blood loss (Chapter 9).

HERNIATION: ("HER-nee-AY-shun") a life-threatening event that occurs when severe brain swelling or bleeding begins to compress brain tissue and force the brain down onto the brain stem where vital functions are controlled (Chapter 6).

IABP: (intra-aortic balloon pump) a device that is placed into an artery in the groin, then advanced into the aorta in the chest. The "balloon-pump" works by balloon inflation and deflation. The goal of this device is to assist the heart in providing adequate blood circulation in cardiogenic shock.

ICP: (intracranial pressure) pressure within the skull (Chapter 6).

ICP MONITOR: a device that monitors pressures within the skull. One way to place an ICP monitor is by performing a ventriculostomy ("Ven-TRICK-you-LOST-ummy") (Chapter 6).

ICU: intensive care unit (preface).

IDIOPATHIC PULMONARY FIBROSIS: a disease of the lungs associated with scar formation and hardening of lung tissue of unknown cause (Chapter 4).

INCENTIVE SPIROMETER: a small handheld apparatus with a mouthpiece that helps a patient practice taking deep breaths to help avoid pneumonia or atelectasis (Chapter 4).

INFARCTION: ("in-fark-shun") a condition that occurs when inadequate blood flow to an organ progresses to a point where there is damage to the organ. For example, a myocardial infarction is damage to the heart muscle, or "heart attack." Brain cell damage is referred to as a CVA or stroke (Chapters 5 and 6).

INTENSIVIST: a physician who has received specialized training in treating critically ill patients. These physicians are often pulmonologists as well, however, physicians with other backgrounds may also have these qualifications.

INTRACEREBRAL HEMATOMA: a hematoma that is located within the brain tissue itself (Chapter 6).

INTRODUCER: a large bore central line that is placed into a large vein in order to allow a pulmonary artery catheter or pacemaker wire to be guided inside it (Chapter 2).

ISCHEMIA: ("iss-KEE-me-uh") inadequate blood supply to any organ that precedes actual infarction (Chapters 5,6).

ITP OR IDIOPATHIC THROMBOCYTOPENIC PURPURA: a disease characterized by antibodies that are produced by the body that destroy platelets and therefore cause low platelet counts (Chapter 10).

IV: (intravenous) a small flexible plastic tube or "catheter" is inserted into the veins of the arms to provide fluid, medication, nutrition, and blood products (Chapter 2).

IV POLE: a pole that holds a bag or bottle of fluids or medications that drips into a patient's vein (Chapter 2).

JAUNDICE: ("JAWN-duss") a yellow discoloration of the skin or eyes that results most commonly from liver disease or hemolysis (destruction of red blood cells) (Chapter 8).

J-TUBE: (Jejunostomy tube) a feeding tube that is placed surgically into a portion of the small intestine (Jejunum) (Chapter 2).

KETOACIDOSIS: acids (ketones) that are produced in poorly controlled diabetes accumulate in the blood and cause this condition (Chapter 10).

KIDNEY TRANSPLANT: a normal kidney is removed from a donor and surgically placed into the body of a patient with a diseased kidney (Chapter 7).

KUB: a simple x-ray technique that shows the abdomen, but cannot provide detailed images of organs.

LACTULOSE: a sugar compound that is used to increase the loss of ammonia through the stool (Chapter 8).

LARGE BOWEL OBSTRUCTION: a blockage in the large bowel (Chapter 8).

LIBERATION: the process of "weaning" or removing the ventilator machine from the patient (Chapter 3).

LIVER: a large gland with many important functions that is located in the upper part of the abdomen on the right side (Chapter 8).

LIVER FAILURE: a condition in which the liver no longer functions normally (Chapter 8).

LIVING WILL: the most common advance directive. It tells your doctor, in writing, what you want or do not want if you should become unable to make decisions yourself (Chapter 11).

LOCAL ANESTHESIA: ("an-es-TEEZ-ya") this is a technique that allows physicians to perform a procedure or simple operation without having to take the patient to the operating room and provide general anesthesia. Basically, liquid "numbing" medication is given to the site on the skin or deeper tissues, using a needle and syringe. Sedatives and intravenous pain medications may also be provided (Chapter 2).

LUMBAR DRAIN: a long thin tube that is inserted into the space between the spinal vertebrae of the lower back in order to drain CSF (cerebrospinal fluid) (Chapter 6).

LVAD (LEFT VENTRICULAR ASSIST DEVICE): mechanical pumps that help the heart maintain blood circulation until a donor heart becomes available (Chapter 5).

MAGNESIUM: a mineral needed by the body that can be measured by a blood test (chapter 10).

MECHANICAL VENTILATION: ("ven-ti-LAY-shun") a machine that provides breathing assistance to a patient who is having severe difficulty breathing. Before a ventilator can be provided to a patient, an endotracheal tube or a tracheostomy tube needs to be in place in the patient's airway. Please note that a ventilator machine is a much more complex system than just providing the patient with oxygen. See CPAP, nasal cannula and oxygen mask (Chapter 3).

MEDIAN STERNOTOMY: an incision made on the breastbone that a surgeon uses to open the chest cavity. This incision is commonly used by heart surgeons (Chapter 4).

MICU: medical intensive care unit (preface).

MRI: (magnetic resonance imaging) a complex diagnostic imaging technique that does not use x-rays. Instead, this technology utilizes large magnets to form detailed images of certain organs (Chapter 6).

MUSCULAR DYSTROPHY: ("DIS-tru-fee") an inherited disorder of the muscle, associated with progressive muscular weakness (Chapter 3).

MYASTHENIA GRAVIS: ("MY-a-STEEN-eea") a neurologic disease caused by antibodies that the body produces. These antibodies damage the connection between nerves and muscles, thus causing muscular weakness (Chapter 3).

MYOCARDIAL INFARCTION: commonly called "heart attack," this occurs when a blocked coronary artery no longer allows adequate blood flow, causing damage to the heart muscle (Chapter 5).

NASAL CANNULA: a simple apparatus that provides oxygen to the patient through the nose using two soft nasal "prongs." This system does not however, provide breaths for the patient (Chapter 3).

NEBULIZER (SVN OR SMALL VOLUME NEBULIZER): a small machine that forces compressed air through a hand-held bulb that allows liquid medications to become a mist that is then breathed in by the patient. Although it is a "breathing machine," it is not a ventilator machine that actually breathes for the patient (Chapter 4).

NEPHROLOGIST: a physician who specializes in the diagnosis and non-surgical treatment of diseases of the kidney.

NEUROLOGIST: a physician who specializes in the diagnosis and non-surgical treatment of diseases of the brain and spinal cord.

NEUROSURGEON: a physician who specializes in the surgical treatment of diseases of the brain and spinal cord.

N-G TUBE: (nasogastric tube) a small feeding tube placed into a nostril and then advanced down the esophagus (swallowing tube) into the stomach (Chapter 2).

NICU: neurological or neurosurgical intensive care unit (preface).

NUCLEAR SCANS: procedures that produce images of the heart by using safe doses of radioactive tracers (Chapter 5).

O-G TUBE: (orogastric tube) same principal as the N-G tube except the tube is started in the mouth (Chapter 2).

ORGAN DONATION: a normal organ is removed from the body of an individual so that it can be surgically placed into the body of another individual whose organ is severely diseased (Chapter 11).

ORGAN TRANSPLANT: a person with a diseased organ has it surgically removed and replaced with a normal organ (donor organ) (Chapter 11).

OXIMETRY: ("ox-IM-it-tree") The act of painlessly estimating blood oxygen levels with a probe on the finger or ear lobe which is then connected to an oximeter machine that displays the oxygen level as a percent of hemoglobin saturation. For example, a reading that is 90% or higher is "better" than a reading that is below 90% (chapter 3).

OXYGEN MASK: a plastic mask that is placed over the mouth and nose that gives the patient different amounts of oxygen. The mask does not however, "breathe" for the patient (Chapter 3).

PANCREATITIS: inflammation of the pancreas that occurs when the body's own digestive enzymes start to inflame the pancreas (Chapter 8).

PARALYTICS: ("pear-a-LIT-ticks") intravenous medications that are given in the ICU on a temporary basis to some patients on the ventilator in order to keep their muscles from moving, thus keeping the patient's own breathing muscles from working against the ventilator.

PARAPLEGIA: ("PEAR-a PLEE-ja") paralysis of the legs and lower part of the body (Chapter 6).

PEG TUBE: a type of G-tube that is placed using an endoscope (Chapter 2).

PERITONEAL DIALYSIS: ("pear-a-ton-EE-al dye-AL-iss-is ") a dialysis technique that uses the lining of the abdomen (peritoneum) as a filter for your blood. A soft flexible catheter is placed into the abdominal cavity and a special solution is put in for a few hours, and then drained out carrying unwanted substances (Chapter 7).

PERITONEUM: ("pear-it-uh-NEE-um) the sac or membrane that surrounds the organs within the abdominal cavity (Chapter 8).

PERITONITIS: infection, irritation, or inflammation of the peritoneum (Chapter 8).

pH: refers to the amount of acid or alkali in the blood, measured by an arterial blood gas sample (ABG) (Chapter 3).

PIGGYBACK: refers to a bag of liquid medications that is attached to an intravenous line that is already in place putting fluid into a patient's vein (Chapter 2).

PLEURAL CAVITY: space between the lung and the rib cage (Chapter 4).

PLEURAL EFFUSION: ("ef-YOU-shun") a collection of abnormal fluid in the pleural cavity (Chapter 4).

PNEUMOTHORAX: ("new-mo-THOR-ax") a condition that occurs when air leaks into the space between the lung and the rib cage (Chapter 4).

PNEUMONIA: ("new-MOAN-ya") pneumonia is an infection that occurs in one or both lungs, and usually is associated with an abnormal chest X-ray (Chapters 3 and 4).

POTASSIUM: a salt/mineral needed by the body that can be measured by a blood test (chapter 10).

PSDA: (Patient Self–Determination Act) a law that gives all legally competent adults the right to make decisions today about the limits of health care treatment they would want to receive in the future if they became unable to communicate their wishes themselves (chapter 11).

PULMONARY: refers to the lungs.

PULMONARY ARTERIES: blood vessels that carry blood with low oxygen levels leave the right side of the heart and enter the lungs in order to gain oxygen and lose carbon dioxide (Chapter 4).

PULMONARY ARTERY CATHETER: see "Swan-Ganz" catheter.

PULMONARY EDEMA: ("PULL-muh-NA-ry eh-DEE-ma") a condition that occurs when fluid enters the lungs, often due to congestive heart failure (CHF), however, can also occur from other causes as well (Chapter 4).

PULMONARY EMBOLUS: ("EM-bowl-us") a condition that occurs when a blood clot travels from the veins in the legs or pelvis to the pulmonary arteries of the lungs (Chapters 3 and 4).

PULMONOLOGIST: a physician who has received specialized training in the diagnosis and non-surgical treatment of lung diseases.

PULSE OXIMETRY: see OXIMETRY

PRESSORS: a term used to describe a class of strong intravenous medications that constrict blood vessels and/or improve the pumping action of the heart in order to increase blood pressure when a patient is in shock (Chapter 9).

PRIMARY PULMONARY HYPERTENSION (PPH): a disease of unknown cause associated with a persistent increase in pressure in the pulmonary arteries (blood vessels) (Chapter 4).

PTCA: see ANGIOPLASTY

QUADRIPLEGIA: "KWOD-ri-PLEE-ja" paralysis of all four limbs (Chapter 6).

RADIOLOGIST: a physician who specializes in reading x-rays and performing procedures in the x-ray department.

RADIOLOGY: the field of medicine that is associated with x-rays, ultrasound, CT scans and MRI tests.

RECTUM: the farthest portion of the large bowel that ends at the anus (Chapter 8).

RENAL FAILURE: ("REE-nul") another name for kidney failure (Chapter 7).

RESPIRATORY FAILURE: any condition that causes the lungs to fail to provide adequate oxygen and ventilation for the body. Commonly, these patients require large amounts of oxygen supplementation, and often need a ventilator machine. While lung diseases such as COPD, ARDS, and pneumonia are possible causes of respiratory failure, other conditions that don't directly affect the lungs may cause respiratory failure as well, for example, sepsis, DKA, neurologic disorders or drug overdose (Chapter 4).

RESPIRATORY RATE: a vital sign that is indicates how fast a person is breathing (Chapter 1).

RESPIRATORY THERAPISTS: these are skilled non-physician staff members who are trained to set up and monitor the ventilator for physicians, provide inhaled medications to improve a patient's breathing, provide oxygen as necessary, and assess the individual's breathing needs.

SEPSIS: a severe infection that often infects the bloodstream (and so the whole body), and may result in shock. (Chapter 9).

SEPTIC SHOCK: shock caused by a severe infection that often infects the blood stream (Chapter 9).

SHOCK: a condition that occurs when a severe abnormality has caused the circulatory system to fail to provide adequate support to organs and cells. Shock is usually associated with low blood pressure, fast heart rate and breathing, acid blood, decreased urine flow, and reduced alertness. There are many causes, but most common are sepsis, heart failure, and blood loss. (Chapter 9).

SICU: surgical intensive care unit (Preface).

SKULL FRACTURES: fractures of the skull bone (Chapter 6).

SPLEEN: a large gland that is situated in the upper part of the abdominal cavity on the left side (Chapter 8).

SPINAL CORD: a large bundle of nerves that transmits electrical signals from the brain to the body. It is surrounded by rings of bone called vertebrae (Chapter 6).

SPINAL CORD INJURY: any injury to the spinal cord (Chapter 6).

STOMACH: a digestive organ that receives food and liquids from the esophagus (swallowing tube) (Chapter 2).

SUBARACHNOID HEMORRHAGE: ("sub-a-RAK-noid-HEM-or-ij") bleeding that is spread thinly over the surface of the brain, inside the skull (Chapter 6).

SUBDURAL HEMATOMA: ("sub-durul-heema-tome-uh") a blood clot between the dura (thick membrane surrounding the brain) and the surface of the brain (Chapter 6).

"STAT": a word used in the hospital for "quick" or "right now."

STENTS: see CORONARY STENT.

SUBCLAVIAN LINE: a central line that is placed in the subclavian vein underneath the collar bone (Chapter 2).

"SWAN-GANZ" PULMONARY ARTERY CATHETER: a catheter with a balloon tip that is placed through a central line access. After the catheter is inserted, the balloon is inflated and the catheter is then "floated" by the bloodstream into the pulmonary artery to measure heart pressures and heart "horsepower." As with other types of central lines, this special catheter is placed under local anesthesia (Chapters 2,5,8 and 9).

TACHYCARDIA: ("TACK-e-KAR-dee-a") refers to an abnormally fast heart rate (Chapter 5).

TBI (TRAUMATIC BRAIN INJURY): an injury to the brain caused by an accident (Chapters 3 and 6).

THORACENTESIS: ("THOR-a-sen-TEE-sus") this procedure removes fluid from the pleural cavity by inserting a needle through the skin on the back of the chest into the pleural cavity, allowing fluid to drain out. Local anesthesia is required, and this procedure is simpler than inserting a chest tube (Chapter 4).

THORACOTOMY: ("THOR-uh-KOT-tum-mee") a surgical technique that involves an incision into the chest in order to operate on the lung (Chapter 4).

THROMBOSIS: ("throm-BOE-sis") a blood clot that causes blockage in a blood vessel.

TPN: (total parenteral nutrition, or "hyperal") liquid nutrition that is infused directly into the bloodstream by using a central line (Chapter 2).

TRACHEA: the "windpipe" (Chapter 3).

TRACHEOSTOMY: ("trak-ee-OSS-tu-mee") or "trake" tube is placed surgically using an incision on the front of the neck below the voice box. The tube is placed directly into the windpipe through a hole made in the neck. A tracheostomy can certainly be temporary, and can be removed when the patient is sufficiently recovered to breathe without it (Chapter 3).

TRAUMA: pertains to injuries that occur due to accidents (Chapters 4 and 10).

TTP OR THROMBOTIC THROMBOCYTOPENIC PURPURA: a blood disorder characterized by low platelets, destruction of red blood cells, confusion, slurred speech, weakness, fever, and kidney disease (Chapter 10).

T-TUBE TRIAL: a method of weaning from the ventilator in which the ventilator machine is turned off, and the endotracheal tube is kept in the patient's windpipe, providing only oxygen as the patient breathes on his/her own (Chapter 3).

ULTRASOUND: an imaging technique similar to submarine "sonar" that bounces sound waves off an organ in order to provide a diagnostic image.

UROLOGIST: a surgeon who specializes in treating diseases of the urinary tract.

VARICES: abnormally enlarged veins that are found in the esophagus, usually caused from chronic liver disease. These veins may cause severe bleeding (Chapter 8).

VASCULAR SURGEON: a surgeon who specializes in surgery of blood vessels.

VASOSPASM: abnormal constriction of arteries resulting in a reduction in their diameter (Chapter 6).

VENTILATOR: see MECHANICAL VENTILATION

VENTRICULAR FIBRILLATION: a potentially lethal abnormal heart rhythm that requires immediate treatment with electrical shock. This rhythm causes cardiac arrest (Chapter 5).

VENTRICULAR TACHYCARDIA: a dangerous abnormal heart rhythm that requires treatment either with medications or electrical shock (Chapter 5).

VENTRICULOSTOMY: ("ven-TRICK-you-LOST-um-mee") a narrow, flexible, hollow tube that is placed in the center of the brain in order to monitor brain pressure (ICP) and drain cerebrospinal fluid (CSF) if the pressure increases too much (Chapter 6).

VERTEBRA: one of the bones of the spinal column (backbone) (Chapter 6).

WEANING: the process of getting a patient off a ventilator machine (Chapter 3).

VOLVULUS: a twist or folding of the bowel (Chapter 8).

WHITE BLOOD CELL COUNT (WBC): a common blood test that measures white blood cells in the blood. High levels often, but not always, indicate infection (Chapter 9).